Self-Assessment in

CLINICAL
HEMATOLOGY

J. A. Holmes
University of Wales College of Medicine
Cardiff, UK

S. Kinsey
St James's Hospital
Leeds, UK

C. A. Ludlam
Royal Infirmary
Edinburgh, UK

D. K. Webb
Llandough Hospital
Cardiff, UK

J. A. Whittaker
University of Wales College of Medicine
Cardiff, UK

2

ℕ Wolfe

Copyright © 1994 Mosby–Year Book Europe Limited
Published in 1994 by Wolfe Publishing, an imprint of Mosby–Year Book Europe Limited
Printed in Spain by Grafos, S.A. ARTE SOBRE PAPEL
ISBN 0 7234 1917 5

For full details of all Mosby–Year Book Europe Limited titles please write to Mosby–Year
Book Europe Limited, Lynton House, 7–12 Tavistock Square, London WC1H 9LB,
England.

A CIP catalogue record for this book is available from the British Library.

Library of Congress Cataloging-in-Publication Data has been applied for.

Contents

Preface

Clinical Haematology has grown considerably in the last 10–15 years. It has evolved from being primarily a diagnostic discipline in the laboratory and now incorporates the additional significant demands of patient management. The excitement of the subject is this unique combination which is commonly given as its attraction to new recruits. Over the years there have been a number of high-quality books concentrating on morphology and/or additional special diagnostic tests. There have also been excellent texts in the traditional mode.

This book provides a different dimension in the form of a question (often morpho-logically based) and answer, covering both diagnosis and management. This will be of considerable value to those willing to learn more about the discipline and indeed those who know how little they know. By its nature there may be debate about what the correct answers are in terms of patient management, a point which the authors acknowledge.

The book consists of three sections—morphology, data interpretation and grey cases—with the answers provided at the end of each section. Readers are advised to fully answer each part of a question before proceeding to the next section. In this way the maximum benefit can be obtained from the book. Most of the grey cases are based on patients which the authors have treated and therefore provide a realistic scenario. The book has aspirations of being both educational and entertaining—we hope it fulfils both.

J.A. Holmes
A.K. Burnett

Acknowledgements

We are grateful to Dr J. M. Jewsbury of the Liverpool School of Tropical Medicine for supplying the slide for **3** and Mr C. J. Lee, Senior MLSO, University of Wales College of Medicine for supplying the slides for **6**, **12** and **15**. Dr P. Thompson of the Department of Medical Genetics, University of Wales College of Medicine has provided detailed cyto-genetic advice. Our thanks also go to Elizabeth Campbell for her secretarial support.

Abbreviations

FBC	Full blood count	DEB	Diepoxybutane
Hb	Haemoglobin	vWF	von Willebrand's factor
WCC	White cell count	vWD	von Willebrand's disease
MCH	Mean cell haemoglobin	HS	Hereditary spherocytosis
MCHC	Mean cell haemoglobin concentration	G6PD	Glucose 6-phosphate dehydroge-nase
MCV	Mean cell volume	HCL	Hairy cell leukaemia
PT	Prothrombin time	AML	Acute myeloblastic leukaemia
KCCT	Kaolin cephalin clotting time	ALL	Acute lymphoblastic leukaemia
APTT	Activated partial thromboplastin time	CML	Chronic myeloid leukaemia
		CLL	Chronic lymphocytic leukaemia
DIC	Disseminated intravascular coagu-lation	MM	Multiple myeloma
		MDS	Myelodysplastic syndrome
PNH	Paroxysmal nocturnal haemo-globinuria	DAT/DCT	Direct antiglobin test
		DDAVP	Desamino D-arginyl vasopressin
TTP	Thrombotic thrombocytopenic purpura	GvHD	Graft versus host disease
		nrbc	Nucleated red blood cell
HUS	Haemolytic uraemic syndrome		

Morphology cases: questions

Morphology case 1

The blood films (**1, 2, 3**) shown here belong to three medical students A, B, and C, respectively, who have been to different parts of the world on their electives. All three have returned with a pyrexia of unknown origin (PUO).

Questions
a What are the respective diagnoses?
b Can you guess where student A has been?
c Can you guess where student B has been?
d Can you guess where student C has been?

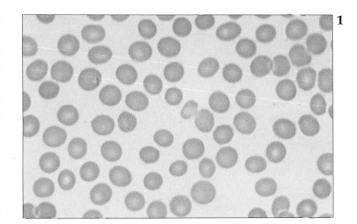

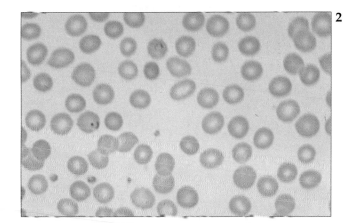

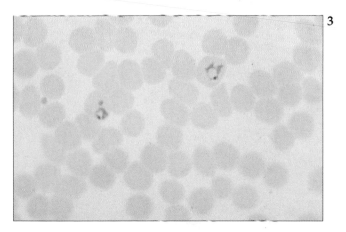

Morphology case 2

A 12-year-old boy presented to his general practitioner with a three week history of anorexia and lethargy. On examination he had a large lower abdominal mass, and the results of a blood count were:

- Hb 6.2 g/dl;
- WCC 3.2 x 10^9/l;
- platelets 78 x 10^9/l.

His bone marrow is shown (4).

Questions

a Discuss the bone marrow appearance. What other diagnostic studies are indicated?

b The bone marrow immunophenotype was CD2 (8%), CD7 (7%), CD10 (66%), CD19 (83%), CD20 (82%), cyt μ (76%), Sm IgM (86%). Discuss the diagnosis.

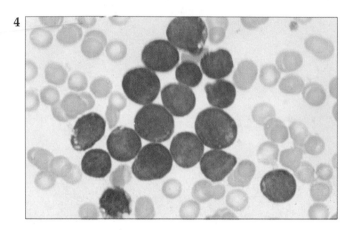

Morphology case 3

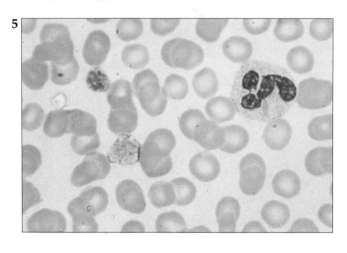

An 81-year-old lady presented with an extensive bruise after excision of a simple mole from her face. Her blood film (5) is shown.

Questions

a What are the abnormalities on the blood film?

b What is the diagnosis?

c What is the mode of inheritance?

d What is the differential diagnosis?

Morphology case 4

A 64-year-old man was admitted as an emergency with shortness of breath. Physical examination revealed signs of cardiac failure. Results of a full blood count were:
- Hb 8.9 g/dl;
- WCC normal;
- platelet count normal.

The peripheral blood film (6) is shown.

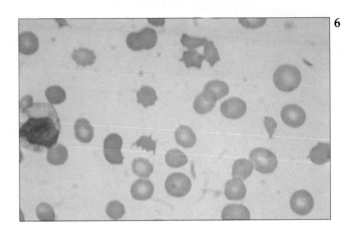

6

Question
What features may lead to a diagnosis?

Morphology case 5

An 84-year-old lady is admitted under the care of the plastic surgeons. A blood sample is received in the haematology laboratory labelled with the clinical details 'unwell'. On investigation:
- Hb is 9.3 g/dl;
- MCV is 83 fl.

Her blood film (7) is shown.

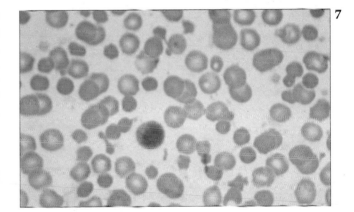

7

Question
What further investigations are required?

Morphology case 6

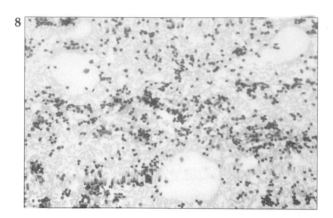

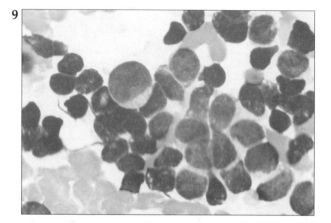

A 3-year-old boy was seen in clinic with unexplained diarrhoea and poor weight gain. Three months later he was pale and tired, and had lost weight. Before hospital admission he developed bilateral proptosis and bone swelling over the right zygoma. A right-sided abdominal mass was palpable. Results of investigations were:

- Hb 6.2 g/dl;
- WCC 8.3 x 10^9/l;
- Platelets 307 x 10^9/l.

Bone marrow slides (**8, 9**) are provided.

Questions
a Discuss the appearances and differential diagnosis.

b Urine VMA/creatinine ratio was 160 mmol/mol (normal less than 9 mmol/mol).What is the diagnosis?

Morphology case 7

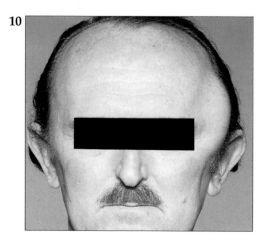

A 53-year-old man presented with a three month history of epistaxis, cough, and difficulty breathing, and a four week history of left temporal swelling (**10**). On examination he had several nasal polyps, and immunoelectrophoresis revealed an IgG paraprotein, 42 g/l.

Questions
a What is the likely diagnosis?

b What is the significance of the paraprotein?

c What treatment should be given?

Morphology case 8

An Asian girl presented at three weeks of age with an umbilical infection not responding to antibiotics from the general practitioner. FBC results were:
- Hb 9.3 g/dl;
- WCC 7.4 x 10^9/l (neutrophils 1%, lymphocytes 87%, monocytes 5%, eosinophils 7%);
- platelets 373 x 10^9/l.

The appearance of a bone marrow aspirate is shown in **11**.

Questions
a What are the main morphological features?
b What is the likely diagnosis?
c What further investigation is needed?

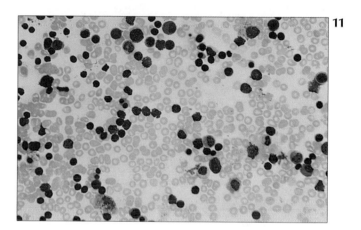

11

Morphology case 9

A 35-year-old woman who has never had surgery attends the Gastroenterology clinic. She has a normal FBC, but her blood film (**12**) is shown.

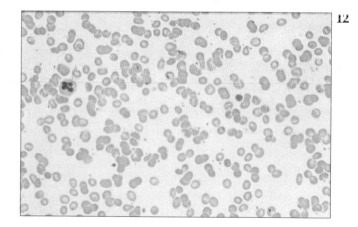

12

Questions
a What abnormalities are illustrated?
b What is the probable diagnosis?

Morphology case 10

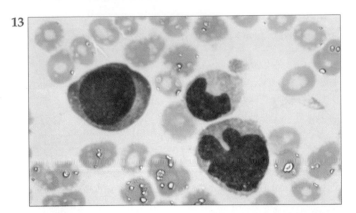

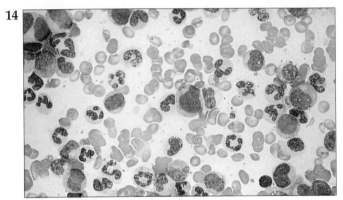

A 1-year-old boy presents with a three month history of weight loss, lethargy, and fever. On examination he has 6 cm splenomegaly. His blood count shows:

- Hb 8 g/dl;
- WCC 29 x 10^9/l;
- neutrophils 14 x 10^9/l;
- monocytes 9 x 10^9/l;
- lymphocytes 4 x 10^9/l;
- metamyelocytes 1 x 10^9/l;
- myelocytes 0.4 x 10^9/l;
- blasts 0.4 x 10^9/l;
- nrbc 0.2 x 10^9/l.

Blood film (**13**) and bone marrow (**14**) slides are provided.

Questions
a What are the features?
b What is the differential diagnosis?

Morphology case 11

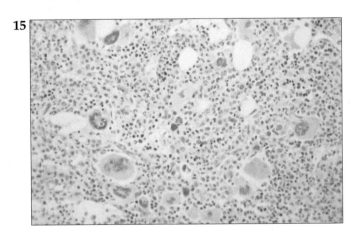

A 45-year-old woman with quiescent seropositive rheumatoid arthritis has persistent thrombocytosis. Blood tests show:

- Hb 8.7 g/dl (MCH 26 pg, MCV 78 fl);
- WCC 8.9 x 10^9/l;
- platelets 860 x 10^9/l;
- ferritin 260 µg/l;
- ESR 45 mm/hour.

A section of trephine biopsy (**15**) is shown.

Question
What do you conclude?

Morphology case 12

A peripheral blood film is shown in **16**.

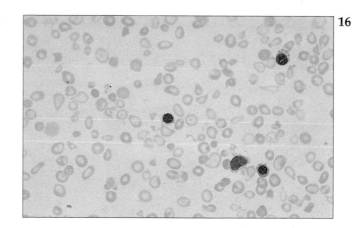

16

Questions
a Describe the main morphological features.
b What is the diagnosis?
c What further investigation is required?

Morphology case 13

A 34-year-old anaesthetist was admitted as an emergency with abdominal pain and bleeding gums. On examination he was mildly jaundiced with tender hepatomegaly and purpura on both legs. FBC revealed:
- Hb 13.6 g/dl;
- WCC 17.6 x 10^9/l;
- platelets 30 x 10^9/l.

His blood film (**17**) is shown.

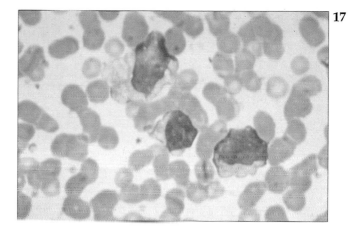

17

Questions
a What is the differential diagnosis?
b What further tests would you perform?
c What is the treatment?

Morphology case 14

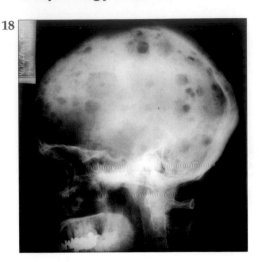

18

The lateral skull radiograph of a 56-year-old man who had complained of backache for six months is shown in **18**.

Questions
a What is the most likely diagnosis?
b What neurological problems may occur in this condition?
c What are the most important prognostic factors?

Morphology case 15

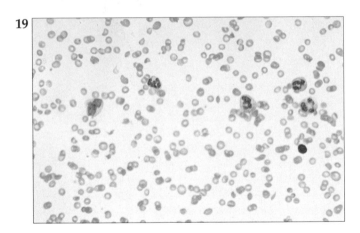

19

A 25-year-old woman was admitted as an emergency with fever and repeated epileptic episodes, which rapidly progressed to a coma. Purpura were noted and a CNS bleed was suspected. FBC revealed:
- Hb 9.4 g/dl;
- WCC 15.8 x 10^9/l;
- platelets 45 x 10^9/l.

The blood film (**19**) is shown.

Questions
a What does the blood film show?
b What diagnosis do you suggest?

Morphology case 16

A 14-year-old girl presented with a two week history of diarrhoea and vomiting. On examination she was feverish (39°C), and had bilateral subconjunctival haemorrhages, pallor, petechiae, and 4 cm hepatomegaly. On investigation:

- Hb 10.6 g/dl;
- WCC 94 x 10^9/l;
- platelets 35 x 10^9/l.

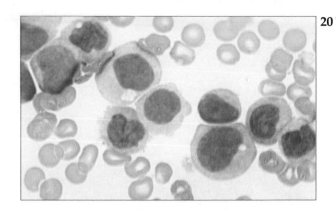

20

Blood film (**20**) and bone marrow (**21**) are shown. Marrow immunophenotype was CD2 (2%), CD7 (13%), CD10 (1%), CD19 (3%), CD33 (83%), CD13 (45%), CD11 (70%), CD14 (55%), CD15 (11%), and HLA-Dr (85%).

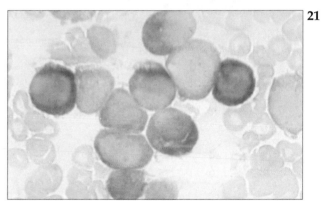

21

Question
Describe and discuss the findings.

Morphology case 17

A 21-year-old woman saw her general practitioner with bruising on her legs. FBC reveals:

- Hb 12.4 g/dl;
- WCC 4.5 x 10^9/l;
- platelets 21 x 10^9/l.

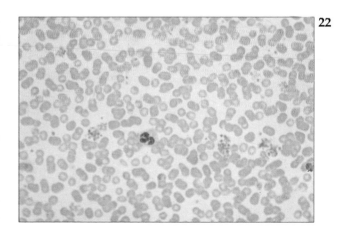

22

Her blood film (**22**) is shown.

Question
A diagnosis of ITP was suspected. What should be done next?

Morphology case 18

23

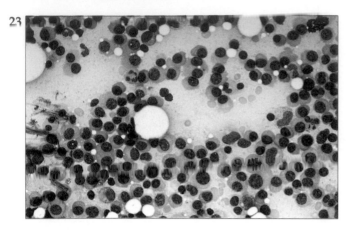

A 60-year-old man presents with a one week history of failing vision and pain in the extremities. **23** shows a bone marrow aspirate.

Questions

a What is the diagnosis?
b What is the correct treatment for the visual disturbance?

Morphology case 19

24

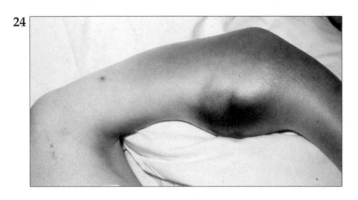

A 5-year-old girl has a large haematoma of her left elbow (**24**), and a lifelong history of easy bruising and epistaxis.

Questions

a What is the differential diagnosis?
b How should the haemarthrosis be treated?

Morphology case 20

25

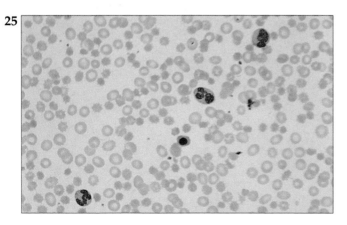

A peripheral blood film is shown in **25**.

Questions

a What are the main morphological features shown?
b What is the probable diagnosis?
c What further investigations are required?

Morphology case 21

A 6-month-old girl was referred for investigation of pancytopenia, first detected at five months. She was previously well and normally grown. On examination she was alert and pale, with hepatosplenomegaly. A blood count showed:

- Hb 7 g/dl;
- WCC 2 x 10^9/l (neutrophils 0.5 x 10^9/l);
- platelets 50 x 10^9/l;
- reticulocyte count 2%.

She was one of three children, with healthy sisters, aged three and six years old. A bone marrow was performed and slides (26, 27) are provided.

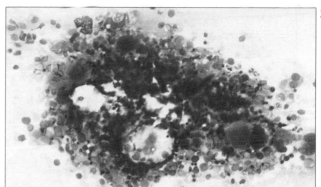

26

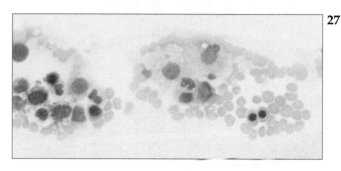

27

Questions

a What are the abnormalities?

b What is the differential diagnosis?

c She developed fever (39°C) and bruising. A coagulation screen showed:

- PT 20/13 secs;
- KCCT 50/40 secs;
- TCT 18/13 secs;
- fibrinogen 0.8 g/dl;
- platelets 20 x 10^9/l.

Liver function tests showed:

- AST 200 iu/l;
- gamma GT 310 iu/l;
- bilirubin 20 µmol/l;
- albumin 25 g/l.

What do these these changes signify?

d What management is recommended?

e A lumbar puncture performed during an infection screen showed:

- WCC 40/mm³ (monocytes 20%, lymphocytes 80%);
- red cells 0;
- protein 1 g/l;
- CSF glucose 4 mmol/l.

Comment on these findings.

f What further investigations would support the diagnosis in this child? What are the treatment options?

Morphology case 22

28

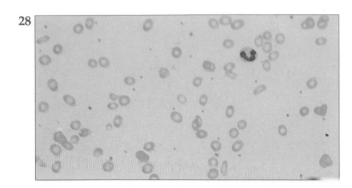

29

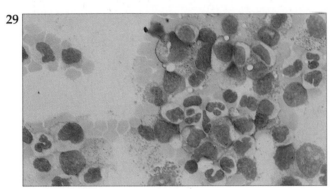

A 13-month-old girl presented with tiredness. Results of a FBC were:
- Hb 2.4 g/dl;
- MCV 79 fl;
- MCH 26.7 pg;
- WCC 5.8 x 10^9/l (neutrophils 1.9 x 10^9/l, lymphocytes 3.3 x 10^9/l, monocytes 0.3 x 10^9/l);
- platelets 369 x 10^9/l.

A peripheral blood film (28) and bone marrow aspirate (29) are shown.

Questions
a What are the main morphological features?
b What is the probable diagnosis?
c What further investigations are required?

Morphology case 23

30

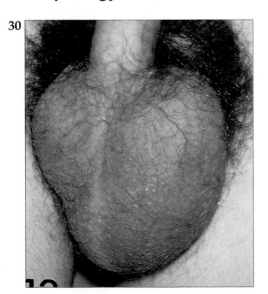

A 14-year-old boy presented with testicular swelling (30) and complains of tiredness for two months. FBC showed:
- Hb 8.0 g/dl;
- WCC 20 x 10^9/l;
- neutrophils 3.4 x 10^9/l;
- blasts 8.6 x 10^9/l;
- platelets 110 x 10^9/l.

Questions
a What is the most likely diagnosis?
b Which other clinical sites might show disease?

Morphology case 24

A 56-year-old lady presented with extensive bruising (31) for the previous four weeks. She had also suffered repeated epistaxis and haematomas for a fortnight, but otherwise felt well. A coagulation screen was as follows:
- platelet count 275×10^9/l;
- APTT 98 secs (normal range 32–40 secs);
- prothrombin time 14 secs (normal range 12–15 secs);
- fibrinogen 3.6 g/dl (normal range 1.5–4.0 g/dl).

Questions
a What is the most likely diagnosis?
b What further investigations are appropriate?
c How should the patient be treated?

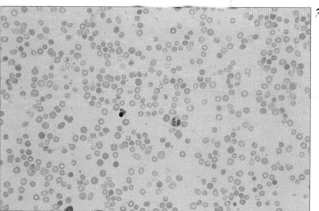

31

Morphology case 25

A peripheral blood film is shown in 32.

Questions
a Describe the main morphological features.
b What is the probable diagnosis?
c What further investigations are required?

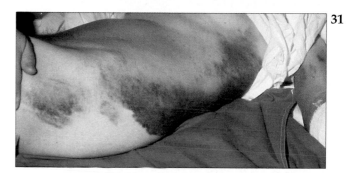

32

Morphology case 26

An 11-year-old girl presented with a three month history of tiredness, pallor, and weight loss. She had previously been well. There was no relevant family history. On examination she was thin and pale with no other abnormal findings. A chest radiograph showed a posterior mediastinal mass. Her blood count showed:

- Hb 10 g/dl;
- WCC 4 (neutrophils 1.8) x 10^9/l;
- platelets 120 x 10^9/l.

Her blood film (33) and a bone marrow aspirate (34) are provided.

Questions

a Describe the findings and further necessary investigations on the bone marrow aspirate.

b Comment on the immunophenotype of the abnormal cells: CD3⁻; CD19⁻; CD10⁻; CD45⁻.

c Marrow cytogenetics revealed an abnormal karyotype 46XX t(2;13). What is the significance of this abnormality?

33
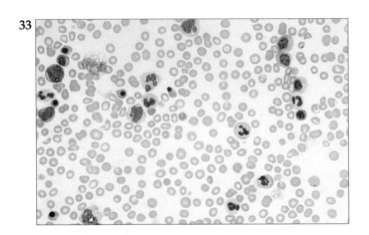

34
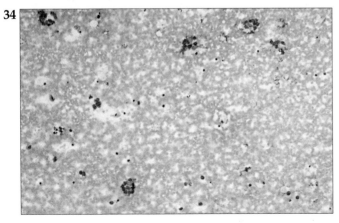

Morphology case 27

A 26-year-old man presented with a 10 week history of recurrent infection and bleeding. Cells from the bone marrow aspirate (**35**) are positive for CD13, CD33, and CD34, but negative for CD10, CD14, CD15, CD19, and TdT.

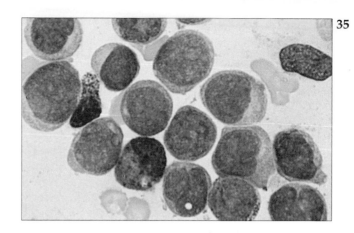

35

Questions

a What is the diagnosis?

b What might deletion of the long arm of chromosome 5 or monosomy 7 indicate?

Morphology case 28

A 27-year-old woman presented with a pruritic clustered rash on her buttocks, knees, and elbows. She was treated successfully, but three months later a FBC showed:

- Hb 10.2 g/dl;
- reticulocytes 120x10^9/l;
- normal WCC;
- normal platelets.

The blood film is shown (**36**).

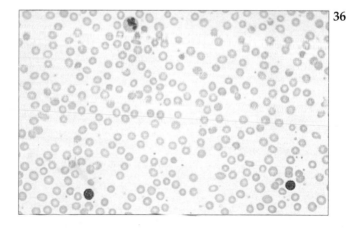

36

Questions

a Comment on the likely course of events.

b Is further intervention required?

Morphology case 29

An 8-year-old boy was referred to clinic with a two year history of anaemia. On examination he was normally grown, and the only abnormal finding was bilateral cryptorchidism. Blood count showed:

- Hb 7 g/dl (MCV 106 fl);
- WCC 3 x 10^9/l (neutrophils 0.5 x 10^9/l);
- platelets 25 x 10^9/l.

A bone marrow was performed, and slides (37, 38) are provided.

Questions

a What is the differential diagnosis?
b What further investigations are required?
c Investigations showed:
- HbF 5%;
- Ham's test negative;
- vitamin B$_{12}$ 224 ng/l;
- folate 4.7 µg/l;
- lymphocyte stress test—an increase in chromosomal breaks and rearrangements following incubation with DEB.

Discuss these results and further management of this child.

37
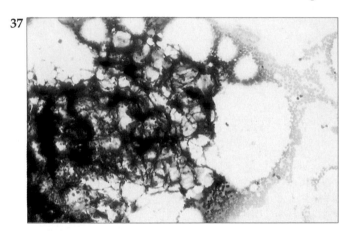

38
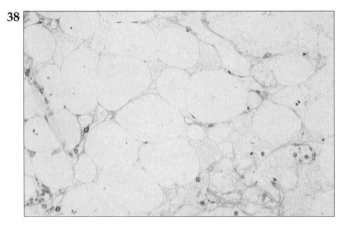

Morphology case 30

A 68-year-old woman is referred to the Out-patient Department by her general practitioner with a presumptive diagnosis of pernicious anaemia. A FBC showed:

- Hb = 8.6 g/dl (MCV 115 fl);
- WCC = 4.4 x 10^9/l;
- platelets 121 x 10^9/l.

The blood film (39) is shown and is reported as showing rouleaux.

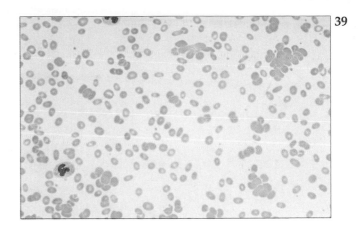

39

Question
What would you do next?

Morphology case 31

A 46-year-old woman presents with a skin rash. The blood count shows:

- Hb 6.8 g/dl;
- WCC 210 x 10^9/l;
- platelets 22 x 10^9/l.

The appearance of her gums (40) is shown.

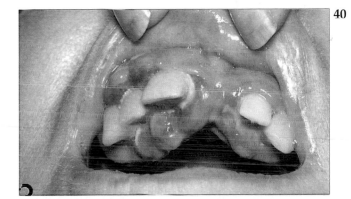

40

Questions
a What is the diagnosis?
b What are the cyto-genetic changes that might indicate a good prognosis?
c What extra treatment would you consider?

Morphology case 32

41

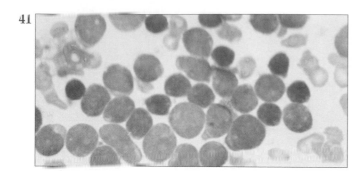

A 4-month-old girl presented with a one week history of malaise and rash. She was the only child of healthy parents. Her past history was unremarkable.

On examination she had a purpuric rash, fever (38°C), lymphadenopathy, and 5 cm hepatosplenomegaly. A blood count showed:

42

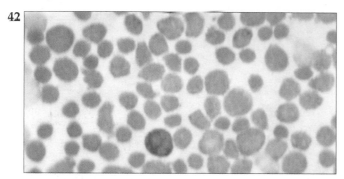

- Hb 4 g/dl;
- WCC 250 x 10^9/l;
- platelets 40 x 10^9/l.

Her blood film (**41**) and marrow cytochemistry (**42**—Sudan black; **43**—PAS) are shown.

43

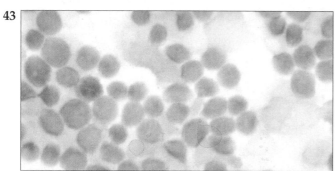

Questions

a What is the diagnosis?

b Marrow cytogenetics showed a clone characterised by 46XX t(9;11). Cell markers were CD19 80%, CD10 5%, CD2 2%, Tdt 70%, Cyt IgM 2%. What is the significance of these findings? What is the approach to treatment and what is the prognosis?

44

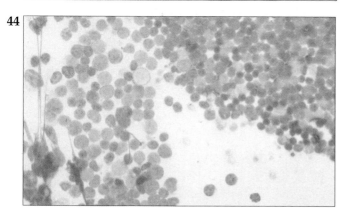

c Two months into treatment she had a routine lumbar puncture. The cytospin (**44**) is provided. What changes are present? What further investigations are indicated and what treatment would you recommend?

Morphology case 33

A 6-year-old girl attended Casualty with a two week history of dyspnoea and cough.

Examination revealed a 2 cm diameter lymph node in the right anterior cervical region, and respiratory distress. The blood count was unremarkable.

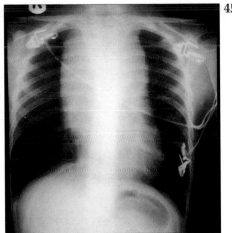

45

Questions
a Discuss the chest radiograph (45), and lymph node section (46) provided.
b What further investigations are indicated?

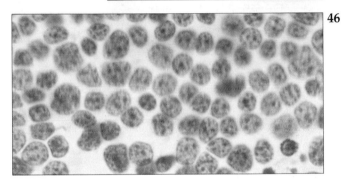

46

Morphology case 34

A 10 year old boy recovering from cytotoxic therapy for acute myeloid leukaemia has a persistent swinging fever and a very slow WCC recovery. 47 shows a bone marrow aspirate.

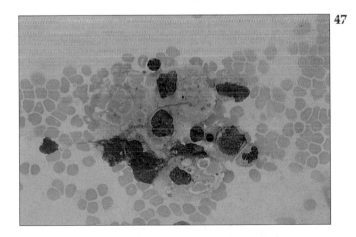

47

Questions
a What is the main morphological feature?
b What is the probable cause for poor count recovery?

Morphology case 35

An 8-year-old girl presented with a three week history of tiredness, pallor, and bone pain. Past medical history was unremarkable. On examination she had generalised lymphadenopathy and 3 cm hepatosplenomegaly. Her blood count showed:

- Hb 9 g/dl;
- WCC 3 x 10^9/l (neutrophils 1x 10^9/l);
- platelets 30 x 10^9/l.

Her bone marrow aspirate is shown (48).

Questions

a What is the probable diagnosis? What other two investigations would you perform on the bone marrow?

b The immunophenotype of the abnormal cells was CD10⁻, CD19⁺, CD22⁺, CD3⁻, SmIg⁺. Comment on these findings.

c Cytogenetics revealed an abnormal clone, 46,XX, t(8;14). Comment on this finding. What are the therapeutic options for this patient?

48
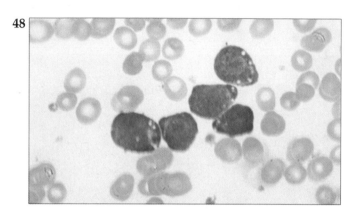

Morphology case 36

49
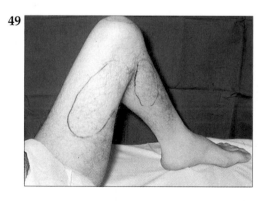

A 35-year-old man with haemophilia presented with pain in the right inguinal region. He preferred to lie with his hip flexed (49), and noted paraesthesia, which have been marked, in parts of his lower limb.

Questions

a What is the differential diagnosis?

b What further investigations may be useful?

Morphology case 37

A peripheral blood film is shown in **50**.

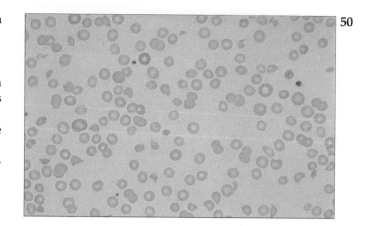

50

Questions

a What are the main morphological features shown?

b What are the probable diagnoses?

c What further investigations are required?

Morphology case 38

A baby presents with a deformity of both upper limbs (**51**) with the radiological features shown in **52**. Some superficial skin bruising is noted.

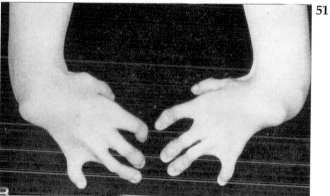

51

Questions

a What is the condition?

b What are the haematological features of this condition?

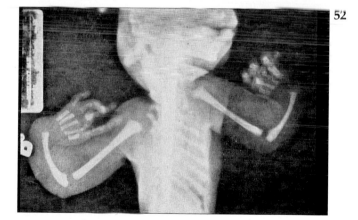

52

Morphology case 39

53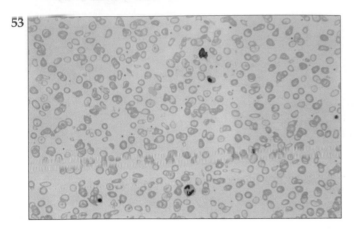

A peripheral blood film is shown in **53**.

Questions
a Describe the main morphological features.
b What is the probable diagnosis?
c What further investigations are required?

Morphology cases: answers

Morphology case 1

a All three students have malaria.

b Student A has *Plasmodium falciparum* with a low degree of parasitaemia. A single ring form can be identified. This ring form is delicate, relatively small, and seen at the edge of the cell. She has been to Kenya.

c Student B has *P. ovale* and has been to West Africa. This form of malaria may be identified by the presence of large coarse ring forms with a single chro-matin dot within a cell with fimbri-ated edges. Most *P. ovale* infections seen in the UK originate in West Africa.

d Student C has *P. vivax*. The ring forms are large with a single chromatin dot. Schüffner's dots are often present and the red cell is usually enlarged. Travellers who return to the UK with *P. vivax* have most commonly visited India.

Morphology case 2

a The bone marrow shows a uniform population of blasts with basophilic, vacuolated cytoplasm (L3 by the FAB classification). Further studies should include marrow immunophenotype and cytogenetics.

b The immunophenotype indicates that the abnormal cells are mature B lymphoblasts. The CD10 positivity (common ALL antigen) is an unusual feature, and would be expected to be absent in most cases of mature B cell disease. The presence of an abdomi-nal mass suggests a diagnosis of stage IV B cell lymphoblastic lymphoma.

Morphology case 3

a The film shows giant platelets and the polymorph contains a Döhle body in-clusion.

b This patient has the May–Hegglin anomaly.

c Dominant.

d Giant platelets are also a feature of the Bernard–Soulier syndrome in which aggregation with ristocetin and Döhle bodies are absent. The May–Hegglin anomaly must be distinguished from idiopathic thrombocytopenic purpura and other congenital thrombocytope-nias, especially those associated with large platelets (e.g. Mediterranean macrothrombocytosis).

Morphology case 4

The blood film shows red cell fragments, which in this case is most likely to indicate a diagnosis of heart valve haemolysis. This man had in fact developed a leaking prosthetic valve and after stabilisation of his cardiac failure, required valve replacement. Red cell fragments may also be seen in association with microangiopathic haemolytic anaemia.

Morphology case 5

The blood film shows red cell fragments and microspherocytes, and the differential diagnosis includes autoimmune haemolytic anaemia, microangiopathic haemolytic anaemia, and hereditary spherocytosis. It would be advisable in such a case to find out more clinical details. This elderly lady had in fact been admitted to the Plastics and Burns Unit with severe burns following a domestic fire resulting in haemolytic anaemia and spherocytes.

Morphology case 6

a The marrow is heavily infiltrated by sheets and clumps of malignant cells. The clinical features and clumping of malignant cells in the marrow suggest metastatic non-haemopoietic tumour.

b The high VMA/creatinine ratio indicates that this tumour is a neuroblastoma.

Morphology case 7

a Extramedullary (soft tissue) plasmacytoma (EMP).These are uncommon tumours of the tissues of the upper respiratory tract, especially the nasopharynx, nasal cavity, and paranasal sinuses, and less commonly the gastrointestinal tract. About 75% of patients are men. The diagnosis can only be established histologically.
b At this level, the paraprotein suggests spread of the disease to bone marrow. Spread, usually to bone, occurs in about 40% of patients; most often this is a single osteolytic lesion, but about 15% have multiple bone deposits or bone marrow plasmacytosis. Radiological spread to bone is unlike that seen in multiple myeloma (MM); bony lesions are usually large and well-circumscribed with no particular predilection for the axial skeleton.
c Chemotherapy as for multiple myeloma.When disease is localised, radiotherapy is the treatment of choice. Prognosis for EMP is excellent when disease is localised, but similar to that for MM if disease has spread to bone.

Morphology case 8

a The main morphological features in the marrow are an absence of neutrophil precursors and absence of mature neutrophils.

b The diagnosis is severe congenital neutropenia (Kostmann's syndrome). The differential diagnosis includes alloimmune neutropenia, caused by passive transfer of IgG anti-neutrophil antibodies from the maternal circulation while *in utero*, and cyclical neutropenia.

c Further investigations required are as follows.

• Monitor peripheral white count and neutrophil count to determine a cyclical nature and to assess spontaneous recovery.

• Anti-neutrophil antibody assay from both maternal and baby's serum to exclude alloimmune neutropenia.

• The parents should have full blood counts to exclude a familial condition.

• Bone marrow should be cultured for CFU-GM, which are reduced in Kostmann's syndrome.

• Marrow and peripheral blood chromosomes analysis to exclude Fanconi's anaemia.

Morphology case 9

a The blood film demonstrates target cells, multiple Howell–Jolly bodies and a giant platelet.

b These features indicate splenectomy or hyposplenism and the most likely diagnosis is splenic atrophy associated with coeliac disease. Other possibilities include ulcerative colitis and Crohn's disease, which are more rarely associated with splenic atrophy.

Morphology case 10

a The blood film shows bizarre monocytes, and the bone marrow an increase in monocytes, with dysplastic changes in the myeloid series (hypogranulation, Pelger-form nuclei).

b The features are those of a juvenile myeloproliferative disorder, in particular juvenile chronic myeloid leukaemia (JCML) or infant monosomy 7 syndrome. Further investigations should include HbF (high in JCML) and marrow cytogenetics.

Morphology case 11

The trephine is hypercellular with multiple pleomorphic megakaryocytes. These features are more consistent with myeloproliferative disease and this lady was assumed to have developed essential thrombocythaemia. Her platelet count was subsequently brought under control with hydroxyurea.

Morphology case 12

a The morphological features demonstrated are hypochromic, microcytic red cells with marked poikilocytosis and some fragmentation. Nucleated red cells are present. There are prominent target cells and some basophilic stippling.
b The diagnosis is β-thalassaemia major.
c Further investigations are:
• Hb electrophoresis, which will show HbF only;

• full red cell genotype (important before starting a transfusion regimen);
• serum ferritin, which is often elevated before transfusion due to increased gastrointestinal uptake of iron;
• screen the parents and family to enable appropriate counselling of individuals and identify potentially 'at risk' pregnancies.

Morphology case 13

a The differential diagnosis includes acute leukaemia, hepatitis, and glandular fever. The blood film is compatible with glandular fever with atypical mononuclear cells. These cells have an amoeboid appearance with coarse chromatin, although nucleoli may be present. The cytoplasm often stains more deeply in the periphery than in the perinuclear area.

b The monospot test, or Paul–Bunnell test was positive. Bone marrow examination showed nonspecific changes.
c There is no specific treatment for glandular fever, although in this case, thrombocytopenia was particularly severe and treatment with corticosteroids may be indicated.

Morphology case 14

a Multiple myeloma.
b Root symptoms from compression fractures; rarely cord compression from vertebral collapse. Peripheral neuropathy (1% of cases) is seen more commonly in osteosclerotic disease and with solitary plasmacytomas.

c Severe anaemia, poor performance rating, renal failure, high β_2 microglobulin levels. Other less important indicators are hypoalbuminaemia, hypercalcaemia, high monoclonal component, and expression of CD10 on plasma cells.

Morphology case 15

a The blood film confirms the thrombocytopenia and neutrophilia, but further inspection reveals fragmented red cells.

b These features are associated with microangiopathic haemolytic anaemia and thrombotic thrombocytopenic purpura (TTP). Subsequent CT scan of the head proved to be normal and TTP was indeed believed to be the diagnosis. The patient subsequently died.

Morphology case 16

The blood film shows large numbers of blast cells with copious pale grey cytoplasm; some with vacuolation and kidney-shaped nuclei. The bone marrow contains similar cells, and dual staining in the combined esterase indicates the presence of both a myeloid and monocytic component.

The immunophenotype indicates acute myeloid leukaemia (lymphoid markers CD2, CD7, CD19, CD10 are negative), with a monocytic component (CD11 and CD14 positivity). The diagnosis is acute myelomonocytic leukaemia (AML M4, FAB classification).

Morphology case 17

The blood film shows the presence of platelet clumps. Modern automated blood cell counters may not discriminate platelet aggregates and will count only those platelets which are unclumped, resulting in a pseudothrombocytopenia. This may be obvious from the 'scattergram,' which the cell counter produces, but blood film examination should be performed where platelet aggregates are most likely to be seen in the tail of the film. A repeat FBC and coagulation screen in this woman proved normal and the diagnosis was presumed to be simple bruising (purpura simplex).

Morphology case 18

a Multiple myeloma with a hyperviscosity syndrome (HVS).

b Immediate plasmapheresis, repeated if necessary, to reduce serum viscosity to less than 4.0 mPascals at which level the clinical side effects of HVS do not occur.

Morphology case 19

a She is likely to have a coagulation factor deficiency rather than thrombocytopenia because haemarthrosis is not a feature of a reduced platelet count or a thrombopathy. The commonest causes of this in a girl would be severe von Willebrand's disease (vWD) or factor XI deficiency. In this instance the factor VIII level was 0.05 iu/ml, vWF ristocetin co-factor activity was less than 0.05 iu/ml, and factor XI level was 0.95 iu/ml. No inhibitor was detectable and a diagnosis of severe vWD is appropriate.

b Factor VIII concentrate should contain vWF of intact multimeric structure (i.e. particularly high molecular weight multimers). During the manufacture of some factor VIII concentrates, particularly those of high purity, the vWF becomes denatured and is of reduced activity in supporting primary haemostasis. It is therefore essential to chose a factor VIII concentrate of proven haemostatic effectiveness in vWD. Desmopressin is inappropriate therapy because the basal vWF level is very low. This drug is usually reserved for patients with type 1 vWD who have basal vWF levels over 0.07–0.10 iu/ml; after desmopressin, the level rises 3–5 fold.

Morphology case 20

a The morphological features are acanthocytes, burr cells, and nucleated red cells.

b These are the features seen in combined hepatic and renal failure. The differential diagnosis includes pyruvate kinase deficiency.

c Further investigations required are:
• renal function tests;
• bilirubin and liver function tests;
• an enzyme assay and family studies to exclude PK deficiency.

Morphology case 21

a The bone marrow is hypercellular, with an increase in megakaryocytes. There is an increase in histiocytes, with haemophagocytosis.

b These changes may reflect a primary histiocytic disorder, or may occur in reaction to systemic illness, particularly autoimmune disease or viral or atypical infection.

c These coagulation abnormalities may reflect either consumption of coagulation factors and platelets (DIC) or impaired production due to liver dysfunction. The fever may be part of the underlying disease process or due to intercurrent infection.

d Management is supportive with co-agulation factor replacement by fresh frozen plasma, cryoprecipitate, and platelet transfusion as indicated clinically. A septic screen is indicated with broad spectrum antibiotic cover pending culture results.

e There is a CSF leucocytosis. These changes do not support bacterial meningitis, but may indicate viral infection. However, the presence of a CSF leucocytosis with lymphocytes and monocytes and high protein, in this clinical context supports a diagnosis of haemophagocytic lymphohistiocytosis (HLH).

f The diagnosis of HLH will be supported by fasting hypertriglyceridaemia, lymphohistiocytic infiltrate of the portal tracts on liver biopsy or a similar infiltrate with haemophagocytosis within lymph node or spleen. A high serum ferritin is a recognised finding in this disorder. Generally there is a very poor prognosis, although responses may be achieved with etoposide, steroids, and intrathecal methotrexate. Bone marrow transplantation may be effective, and the family should be tissue typed. Given the poor prognosis a matched unrelated donor search is indicated in the absence of a family donor.

Morphology case 22

a The peripheral blood reveals normochromic normocytic red cells. The marrow shows an absence of erythroid precursors.

b The diagnosis is red cell aplasia (Diamond–Blackfan syndrome). Diamond–Blackfan syndrome is associated with low birth weight and other dysmorphic features including short stature, wide-set eyes, limb abnormalities (e.g. triphalangeal thumbs), and renal abnormalities.

c Further investigations include:
• a reticulocyte count and parvovirus B19 titres (parvovirus B19 infection is associated with a transient red cell aplasia; with regular monitoring of Hb and reticulocytes, a transient red cell aplasia can be demonstrated);
• serum iron, ferritin, folic acid, B_{12}, and erythropoietin (all elevated in Diamond–Blackfan syndrome);
• HbF (usually increased in Diamond–Blackfan syndrome);
• marrow culture (which shows reduced BFU-E in Diamond–Blackfan syndrome).

Morphology case 23

a Acute lymphoblastic leukaemia. Presentation with testicular disease is rare, although the testicle is the initial site of relapse in 10–13% of boys.

b Central nervous system and rarely the eye or the kidney.

Morphology case 24

a The APTT indicates a deficiency in the intrinsic part of the coagulation cascade. Factor VIII deficiency is the commonest cause of prolonged APTT in someone who is not systemically unwell or on an anticoagulant. As the history is a recent onset haemorrhagic diathesis, acquired haemophilia is the most likely diagnosis. Individuals with an antiphospholipid antibody do not present with bleeding.

b The APTT should be repeated on a mixture of patient and normal plasma. In acquired haemophilia the APTT on the mixture will remain prolonged due to the presence of an anti-factor VIII antibody inhibiting the factor VIII activity in the normal plasma. Factor VIII level will be markedly reduced. The activity of the antibody should be determined against human and porcine factor VIII. It is important to distinguish this rare inhibitor from the commoner lupus anticoagulant, which may prolong the APTT and is not corrected by normal plasma. This inhibitor is not associated with a haemorrhagic state.

c In a few patients with acquired haemophilia there may be residual factor VIII in the plasma. If the degree of bleeding is relatively slight or follows a minor operation, desmopressin may be effective in securing haemostasis. In the more usual situation the plasma factor VIII level is less than 0.01 iu/ml and it is necessary to give factor VIII concentrate. If the antibody level is low against human factor VIII then treatment should be started with human factor VIII concentrate. In many instances the level is low against porcine factor VIII and it is appropriate to give treatment with porcine factor VIII concentrate. Use of immunosuppressive therapy should be considered; prednisolone and cyclophosphamide are most commonly used. Intravenous immunoglobulin may also be used to suppress the level of the anti-factor VIII antibody.

Morphology case 25

a Features of the peripheral blood film are polychromasia, microspherocytes, and nucleated red cells.

b The diagnosis is hereditary spherocytosis (HS).

c Further investigations required are as follows.

• Osmotic fragility, which will demonstrate increased susceptibility to lysis and will be more pronounced after 24-hour incubation.

• Acidified glycerol lysis test, which will also show increased lysis.

• Red cell membrane SDS-PAGE, which may identify a membrane protein deficiency including ankyrin, β-spectrin or protein 3 defects in autosomal dominant HS. Recessive HS is associated with α-spectrin defects.

• A family study because of the pattern of inheritance.

• Bilirubin and liver enzyme estimations because chronic haemolytic anaemias are associated with an increased incidence of pigment gallstones and gallbladder disease.

Morphology case 26

a The blood film is leucoerythroblastic with nucleated red blood cells, myelocytes, and metamyelocytes. These appearances occur in marrow infiltration (leukaemia, lymphoma, metastatic cancer), myeloproliferative disease, severe haemolysis, osteopetrosis, hypoxia, or infection. The bone marrow shows clumps of primitive mononuclear cells with copious, vacuolated, basophilic cytoplasm. These could be either lymphoblasts or secondary malignancy. The childhood solid tumours with these appearances include neuroblastoma, Ewing's sarcoma, and rhabdomyosarcoma. Further investigations would include cell immunophenotype and cytogenetics.

b These findings are consistent with secondary tumour in the bone marrow. CD3 is a T cell marker, CD19 and CD10 are B lymphoid markers, and CD45 is a panleucocyte marker. All are negative indicating a non-haematological malignancy.

c The t (2;13) is characteristic of alveolar rhabdomyosarcoma and the diagnosis is metastatic rhabdomyosarcoma with intrathoracic primary tumour.

Morphology case 27

a The morphology and the cell markers suggest FAB M1 acute myeloid leukaemia. CD33 is found on myeloid precursors and CD34 on myeloid stem cells. CD13 is a marker for monocyte, but is also found on mature polymorphonuclear neutrophils.

b AML secondary to occupational or mutagen exposure, or AML with preceding MDS.

Morphology case 28

a The blood film shows bite cells, which occur in chronic oxidative intravascular haemolysis. Dapsone prescribed for dermatitis herpetiformis is the likely culprit. If the spleen is intact, a Heinz body preparation may show no Heinz bodies. Functional hyposplenism occurs in dermatitis herpetiformis and a blood film stained with brilliant cresyl blue will reveal Heinz bodies.

b Haemolysis in this case is well compensated and dapsone only needs to be stopped if the patient becomes anaemic.

Morphology case 29

a The patient has pancytopenia, with a macrocytosis. Bone marrow particles are grossly hypocellular, with few remaining haematopoietic cells. The marrow trephine confirms severe hypoplasia, consistent with aplastic anaemia.

b Further investigation of this child would include:

• haematinics;
• full virology (including a hepatitis screen);
• autoantibodies;
• serum immunoglobulins;
• HbF level;
• Ham's test to exclude PNH;
• lymphocyte stress test with DEB for Fanconi's anaemia (Fanconi's anaemia is a possibility as this child has cryptorchidism, a recognised abnormality in this syndrome).

c The investigations show a high HbF, consistent with stress erythropoiesis, normal B_{12} and folate levels, negative Ham's test, but positive lymphocyte stress test. The diagnosis is therefore Fanconi's anaemia, and a clinical history of presentation around 8 years of age, with a preceding falling blood count, is typical for this disorder. Management is by bone marrow transplant from a full-matched family donor if possible, but in the absence of a family donor, an unrelated donor search is indicated. More than 50% of these children respond to androgen therapy and this should be instituted. Complications of androgens include virilisation, and hepatic tumours. Fanconi's anaemia is associated with an increased risk of both leukaemia and cancer. Children successfully treated by transplantation therefore need careful follow-up to detect these associated disorders.

Morphology case 30

The blood film in fact shows cold agglutinins, which should disappear if the blood is warmed to 37°C and the film remade. Automated cell counters will indicate a falsely high MCV where cold agglutinins are present if the blood is assayed at room temperature. B_{12} and folate levels were normal. Direct Coomb's test was positive for complement only. There was no evidence of mycoplasma infection or a lymphoproliferative disorder and this woman was assumed to have idiopathic cold haemagglutinin disease (CHAD).

Morphology case 31

a FAB M4 (or M5) acute myeloid (myelomonocytic) leukaemia.

b inv (16) (p13q22) with an increased number of marrow eosinophils, which are often hypergranular. Other rarer anomalies of chromosome 16 (e.g. del (16) (q22) and t (16;16) (q13;q22) carry a similarly good prognosis.

c CNS prophylaxis with cranial irradiation and intrathecal methotrexate to protect against the higher risk of CNS disease in M4 and M5 AML.

Morphology case 32

a The blood film shows a high white count due to the presence of a monomorphic population of leukaemic blasts. The cytochemistry shows a negative PAS and Sudan black. The likely diagnosis is acute lymphoblastic leukaemia, but immunophenotyping and cytogenetics are indicated to support the diagnosis.

b The immune phenotype indicates early pre-B (NULL) cell ALL. Translocations involving 11q are typical of this disorder. Both the high WCC and age of the child (i.e. less than 1 year) indicate a poor prognosis.

c The CSF cytospin is heavily infiltrated with leukaemic blasts. This may be confirmed by immune phenotype, although this may prove technically difficult on CSF samples. The bone marrow should be examined to exclude medullary relapse. The prognosis after relapse on treatment is poor. As the child is too young to tolerate craniospinal irradiation, treatment is by intrathecal or intraventricular chemotherapy with delayed irradiation at two years of age.

Morphology case 33

a The chest radiograph shows a widened superior mediastinum, due to a mediastinal mass. A lateral chest radiograph is indicated to demonstrate the position of the mass in the mediastinum. The lymph node section shows a uniform infiltrate of small, basophilic cells with prominent nucleoli. The clinical features, and lymph node section suggest a T cell lymphoblastic lymphoma.

b Further investigations include a bone marrow aspirate, and lumbar puncture to exclude bone marrow and CNS disease. Immunocytochemistry on the node sections is required to confirm the diagnosis.

Morphology case 34

a The striking morphological feature is haemophagocytosis. The likely cause is virus-associated haemophagocytic syndrome. This is a benign disorder characterised by histiocytic proliferation with haemophagocytosis associated with a systemic viral infection. The patient is usually pancytopenic and toxic, and after myelosuppressive chemotherapy it may be a cause for delayed count recovery.

b Epstein–Barr virus, cytomegalovirus, herpes simplex, varicella zoster, adenovirus, and parvovirus B19 have all been implicated.

In this case adenovirus infection was the cause of haemophagocytosis and delayed peripheral count recovery.

Morphology case 35

a The marrow is replaced by a uniform population of blasts with prominent nucleoli and basophilic cytoplasm with vacuolation. Although vacuolation may occur in other FAB subtypes, the appearances are suggestive of FAB type L3, which implies mature B cell acute lymphoblastic leukaemia. Further investigations are cell immunophenotyping and cytogenetics.

b The presence of CD19 and CD22 indicates B lineage, and the presence of surface immunoglobulin (SmIg) indicates that these are mature B cells. CD10 is the common ALL marker and is often negative in mature B cell leukaemia. CD3 is a T cell marker and is therefore negative.

c The 8;14 translocation is typical of mature B cell ALL/lymphoma. The therapeutic options lie between chemotherapy alone or, if an appropriate family donor exists, with subsequent allogeneic BMT. Although the prognosis for mature B cell lymphoblastic leukaemia has been particularly poor, current treatment protocols have produced high remission and survival rates. It is therefore appropriate to treat first with chemotherapy alone.

Morphology case 36

a The most probable diagnosis is a haematoma in the psoas. The hip is flexed to reduce the tension in the muscle and limit the pressure on the femoral nerve as it passes under the inguinal ligament. The paraesthetic areas marked on the skin are due to the entrapment of the femoral nerve. The femoral nerve palsy from a severe psoas bleed may result in marked weakness of the quadriceps muscle; following resolution of the haematoma walking may be impaired due to permanent loss of muscle activity. A psoas bleed must be distinguished from a bleed into the hip joint. This usually presents with localised pain in the inguinal region and pain on hip movement. Acute appendicitis must be considered especially if the specific features of a psoas bleed or hip haemarthrosis are absent.

b An abdominal ultrasound will reveal the presence of a psoas haematoma. This investigation is particularly useful for following the resolution of the bleed. Treatment with factor VIII should be continued until the haematoma has completely resolved otherwise it is likely to recur.

Morphology case 37

a The morphological features are marked red cell fragmentation with spherocytes and polychromasia. Platelet numbers are very low. These are the features of a microangiopathic haemolytic anaemia.

b The differential diagnosis must include haemolytic uraemic syndrome (HUS), thrombotic thrombocytopenic purpura (TTP), and disseminated intravascular coagulation (DIC).

c Further investigations required are.
• a coagulation screen and fibrinogen, which will be abnormal in DIC;
• urea and creatinine, which will be abnormal in HUS, and may also be abnormal in TTP;
• urine microscopy and culture;
• an infection screen to identify a possible infective cause precipitating HUS or DIC.

This girl had HUS. Toxin-producing *Escherichia coli*, particularly strain 0157, are implicated in the pathogenesis of HUS.

Morphology case 38

a The child has thrombocytopenia with absent radius (TAR) syndrome.

b Thrombocytopenia is usually recognised as a neonate and within the first few months many have symptoms of thrombocytopenia. The platelet count is usually in the range of 15–30 x 10^9/l. A polymorph leucocytosis is common with a left shift. Bone marrow examination reveals a paucity of megakaryocytes and myeloid hyperplasia. If babies survive the first year of life when the mortality is approximately 30%, the prognosis markedly improves. Transfusions of platelets should be kept to a minimum to avoid alloimmunisation.

Morphology case 39

a The peripheral blood film shows irreversibly sickled cells, microcytic red cells, many target cells, polychromasia, and nucleated red cells.

b The diagnosis is sickle cell disease (Hb SS) with co-inheritance of α-thalassaemia trait. The increased number of target cells is suggestive of α-thalassaemia or Hb SC disease.

c Further investigations would include the following.
- Hb electrophoresis, which showed HbS only.
- Incubation of red cells with brilliant cresyl blue, which may demonstrate HbH bodies and allows detection of α-/α- or αα/-- α-thalassaemia.
- A family study of FBC, electrophoresis, and α/β globin chain synthesis for counselling.

Data interpretation: questions

Data interpretation 1

A 21-year-old man presents with a life-long history of easy bruising, epistaxis as a child, and bleeding for 30 hours after dental extraction. The results of investigations are shown in **54**.

Questions
a What is the diagnosis?
b A molar tooth requires extraction; what haemostatic therapy would be appropriate?

54

Test	Result	Normal
APTT	36 secs	28–38
PT	14 secs	13–16
Fibrinogen	2.3 g/l	1.5–4
Factor VIIIC	0.38 iu/ml	0.50–1.50
vWF antigen	0.32 iu/ml	0.45–1.40
vWF ristocetin co-factor	0.05 iu/ml	0.45–1.35
Bleeding time	12 mins	Up to 8
Platelets	230 x 10^9/l	

Data interpretation 2

Questions
a–f Discuss the significance of the cytogenetic abnormalities in childhood leukaemia listed in **55**.

55

Cytogenetic abnormalities in childhood leukaemia

a t(4;11)(q21;q23)
b t(1;19)(q23;p13)
c t(8;14)(q24;q11)
d Monosomy 7
e t(9;22)(q34;q11)
f t(8;21)(q22;q22)

Data interpretation 3

The conditions listed in **56** are associated with antibody formation.

Questions
a–g What is the usual specificity of the antibodies?

56

Conditions associated with antibody formation

a Treatment with methyldopa
b Paroxysmal cold haemoglobinuria
c Cold haemolytic agglutination disease (CHAD)
d *Mycoplasma* pneumonia
e Post-transfusion purpura
f Rheumatoid arthritis
g Infectious mononucleosis

Data interpretation 4

57

Test	Result
Hb	10.4 g/dl
WCC	123.4 x 10⁹/l (neutrophils13.2 x 10⁹/l, lymphocytes 29.5 x 10⁹/l, monocytes 2.4 x 10⁹/l, atypical lymphoid cells 76.6 x 10⁹/l)
Platelets	67 x 10⁹/l
Bone marrow aspirate	Heavy infiltration with atypical lymphoid cells

Immunophenotype (bone marrow cells)

CD2	9% positivity
CD3	67%
CD4	32%
CD5	37%
CD7	83%
CD8	18%
CD9	8%
CD10	11%
CD11	3%
CD13	2%
CD19	6%
CD20	9%
CD22	2%
CD23	17%

A 22-year-old man presented with a three week history of excessive tiredness. Examination showed generalised multiple shotty lymph nodes, but no other abnormalities. The results of investigations are shown in **57**.

Questions
a What is the diagnosis?
b Which immunophenotyping tests are in keeping with this diagnosis?
c What features suggest that the prognosis is poor?

Data interpretation 5

58

Feature	Patient					
	a	b	c	d	e	f
A1 cells	0	0	3+	0	0	2+
B cells	0	0	3+	3+	3+	3+
O cells	0	0	1+	0	0	0
Anti-A	0	3+	1+	3+	0	3+
Anti-B	0	3+	1+	2+	0	0
O high titre	0	3+	1+	3+	3+	3+
Auto	0	0	1+	0	0	0

Questions
a–f Determine the ABO group of patients a–f (**58**).

Data interpretation 6

A neonate aged two weeks with a respiratory tract infection had a FBC, the results of which were:

- Hb 16.1 g/dl (MCV 99 fl);
- WCC 19.5 x 10^9/l (neutrophils 11.8 x 10^9/l, lymphocytes 3.9 x 10^9/l);
- platelets 524 x 10^9/l.

The H*2 automated cell counter printout is shown in **59**.

```
SEQ#       0000179
TIME       13:28  14/07/93        MORPHOLOGY FLAGS
SYS#       282                  PARAMETER  SUSP  VERIFY
ID         0000000000017          ANISO
           CBC                    MICRO
H 19.45    x10³/L  WBC            MACRO    +
   5.06    x10⁶/L  RBC            VAR
  16.1     g/dL    HGB            HYPO
   .501            HCT            HYPER
H 99.1     fL      MCV            L SHIFT
  31.8     pg      MCH            ATYP     +
  32.1     g/dL    MCHC           BLASTS
H 15.4     %       RDW            OTHER
   2.72    g/dL    HDW            OTHER
H 524      x10³/L  PLT
   7.9     fL      MPV
  53.4     %       PDW            RBC VOLUME
H  .41     %       PCT            (0-200 fL)
RBC FLAGS          0100
           DIFF    x10³/L
  60.6     NEUT H  11.78
  20.0     LYMP     3.89          HGB CONC
   7.0     MONO H   1.36          (0-50 g/dL)
   2.4     EOS       .47
    .6     BASO      .12
H  9.4     LUC  H   1.82
                                  PLT VOLUME
                                  (0-20 fL)
WBC FLAGS          0011
```

Questions

a What abnormality is shown?

b What is the natural history of the disorder?

Data interpretation 7

A 15-year-old boy of West African birth presented with a large lymph node in the left side of his neck. The mass had been present for only three weeks, but was said to be rapidly increasing in size. No other nodes were palpable and the spleen and liver were not clinically enlarged. The results of investigations are shown in **60**.

Questions

a What is the diagnosis?

b What other investigations should be done?

Test	Result
Hb	13.2 g/dl
WCC	8.6 x 10^9/l (normal differential)
Platelets	162 x 10^9/l
Lymph node biopsy	Replacement with large lymphoid cells with foamy cytoplasm containing numerous vacuoles
Cytogenetics on the lymph node	Reciprocal translocation t(8;14)(q24;q32)
Immunophenotype	CD2–; CD3–; CD5–

Data interpretation 8

61

Test	Result
Hb	6.5 g/dl
Red cell indices	Normal
Reticulocytes	15% (300 x 10^9/l)
WCC	8 x 10^9/l
Platelets	250 x 10^9/l
Serum bilirubin	55 μmol/l
DAT anti-IgG	+++
Anti-C3d	Negative

A 10-year-old girl was seen with a two month history of tiredness and pallor. There had been an episode of migratory arthralgia with swelling of her knees. This had improved after several days. Her mother had been treated for nephrotic syndrome 8 years previously. Examination showed a well, normally grown girl with mild jaundice and pallor. Her spleen was palpable 5 cm below the left costal margin. Her joints were normal. The results of investigations are shown in **61**.

Questions
a Discuss the diagnosis and further investigation.
b Discuss the management.

Data interpretation 9

62

Test	Result	Normal
Hb	7.2 g/dl	
WCC	3.1 x 10^9/l	
Platelets	74 x 10^9/l	
Reticulocytes	20 x 10^9/l	
DCT	Negative	
Bilirubin	57 μmol/l	1–17 μmol/l
AST	94 iu/l	5–45 iu/l
Alkaline phosphatase	150 iu/l	30–115 iu/l
Hepatitis B		
e antigen	Negative	
c antigen	Negative	
e antibody	Positive	
c antibody	Positive	
s antigen	Positive	
Hepatitis C antibody	Negative	

A 55-year-old man with myelodysplastic syndrome has become transfusion-dependent in the past six months. He requires a transfusion of four units of packed cells every 6–8 weeks. On attendance at the Outpatient Department six weeks since his last transfusion, he appeared jaundiced. The results of investigations are shown in **62**.

Questions
a What is the probable cause of his jaundice?
b Should his blood be labelled 'high risk'?

Data Interpretation 10

A 32-year-old West Indian man had a haemoglobinopathy screen showing:
- Hb 14.5 g/dl (MCV 93 fl);
- RBC 4.91 x 10^{12}/l;
- HbA2 3.0% (normal 1.6–3.4%);
- HbF less than 1.0 % (normal less than 1.0%).

Hb electrophoresis was performed and the gels are shown in **63** (pH 8.6) and **64** (pH 6.2). The Hbs in the different lanes are lane 1 AA, lane 3 patient, lane 5 AC, lane 6 AS, lane 7 SC, lane 8 AE.

Question
What is the diagnosis?

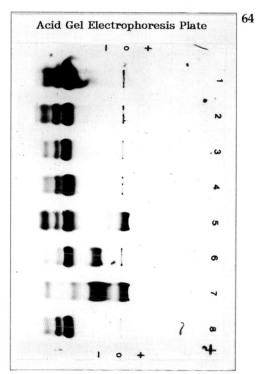

64

Acid Gel Electrophoresis Plate

63

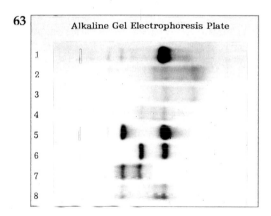

Alkaline Gel Electrophoresis Plate

Data interpretation 11

A 45-year-old man complains to his general practitioner of headaches. He smokes 20 cigarettes a day and drinks 20 pints of beer a week. On examination, he is plethoric and his blood pressure is 150/100 mm Hg. There are no other positive findings. Results of his FBC and blood volume estimations are shown in **65**. A diagnosis of polycythaemia is suspected.

Questions
a Does the patient have polycythaemia?
b Discuss his management.

Test	Result	Normal	65
Hb	18.4 g/dl		
Haematocrit	0.54		
MCV	98 fl		
WCC	9.7 x 10^9/l		
Platelets	184 x 10^9/l		
Red cell mass	34 ml/kg	25–35	
Plasma volume	29 ml/kg	30–40	

Data interpretation 12

66

Test	Result
Hb	8.2 g/dl
WCC	86 x 10^9/l (neutrophils 1.1 x 10^9/l, lymphocytes 3.8 x 10^9/l, blasts 77 x 10^9/l)
Platelets	15 x 10^9/l
Immuno-phenotype	
CD2	3% positivity
CD3	7%
CD5	9%
CD7	4%
CD9	3%
CD11	8%
CD13	57%
CD14	78%
CD15	32%
CD19	11%
CD33	37%
CD34	66%
Karyotyping studies	100% of marrow cells are t(9;22)(q34;q11); 75% of cells contain an additional chromosome 8 and isochromosome (17q)

A 45-year-old man, who had not previously sought medical advice, gave a history of chronic ill health for two years characterised by recurrent bouts of left upper abdominal aching pain. Three days before presentation, he had noticed skin bruises and on the day of admission, he had a spontaneous nose bleed. Examination showed a widespread petechial skin rash and massive splenomegaly. The results of some of the investigations are shown in **66**.

Questions
a What is the diagnosis?
b Which finding do you consider to be most characteristic of this diagnosis?

Data interpretation 13

67

Test	Result	Normal
APTT	40 secs	28–38
PT	14 secs	13–16
Fibrinogen	1.9 g/l	1.5–4.0
Factor VIIIC	0.32 iu/ml	0.5–1.5
vWF antigen	0.75 iu/ml	0.45–1.40
vWF ristocetin co-factor	0.48 iu/ml	0.45–1.35
Platelets	250 x 10^9/l	
Bleeding time (template)	6 mins	Up to 8

A 25-year-old woman bled following tonsillectomy and required three units of blood. There is no other personal or family history suggestive of a bleeding disorder. The results of investigations are shown in **67**.

Questions
a What is the diagnosis?
b How can the diagnosis be confirmed?

Data interpretation 14

A 6-year-old girl presented with pallor and bruising. There were no other abnormalities on examination. The results of investigations are shown in **68**.

Question
a Discuss the diagnosis.
b Discuss the prognosis.
c Discuss the management.

Test	Result	68
Hb	6 g/dl	
Reticulocytes	5 x 10⁹/l	
WCC	3 x10⁹/l (neutrophils 0.6 x10⁹/l, lymphocytes 2.2 x10⁹/l, monocytes 0.2 x 10⁹/l)	
Platelets	80 x 10⁹/l	
Bone marrow aspirate and trephine	Hypocellular, with no increase in blasts	
HbF	4%	
Ham's test	Negative	
Lymphocyte cytogenetics	No increase in breakages after incubation with diepoxybutane (DEB)	

Data interpretation 15

A 68-year-old man presented with a three month history of weight loss and progressive tiredness. For three weeks, he had noticed aching pain in his upper abdomen. Examination showed massive splenomegaly, but apart from skin pallor, there were no other features. Results of investigations are shown in **69**.

Questions
a What is the diagnosis?
b What is the prognosis?

Test	Result	69
Hb	8.4 g/dl	
WCC	384 x 10⁹/l	
Lymphoid cells	365 x 10⁹/l	
Platelets	56 x 10⁹/l	
Blood film	Neutropenia with numerous large lymphoid cells, many having a large single nucleolus	
Bone marrow aspirate	Almost entirely replaced with similar cells	
Immunophenotype	Strong CD22 and CD19 positivity; CD5 and CD10 negative	

Data interpretation 16

The 4-year-old son of Gambian (West Africa) parents was born in the UK and the whole family are migrating back to The Gambia on a permanent basis. At an earlier date when the child had iron deficiency anaemia he was screened for haemolytic problems with a G6PD result of 0.9 iu/g Hb (normal range 6.7–9.9 iu/g Hb). His FBC results are:
- Hb 11.8 g/dl (MCV 90 fl),
- WCC 9.1 x 10^9/l (normal differential);
- platelets 419 x 10^9/l;
- reticulocytes 3.7%.

Questions
a What is the diagnosis?
b What further investigations are required?
c What advice would you give to the family?

Data interpretation 17

70

Test	Result
Hb	7.3 g/dl
WCC	1.2 x 10^9/l (neutrophils 0.3 x 10^9/l, blast-like cells 0.8 x 10^9/l)
Platelets	22 x 10^9/l
Marrow aspirate and trephine	Hypercellular with increased reticulin. Aspirate showed about 30% primitive cells with scanty cytoplasm and dense chromatin. Many cells had cytoplasmic blebs. Moderate trilineage dysplasia
Immuno-phenotype	Strong positivity for CD41
Cytogenetics	Translocation t(3;3)(q21;q26) in all cells examined
Cytochemistry on marrow cells	
Sudan black	Negative
Myeloperoxidase	Negative
PAS	Some fine granular PAS positivity in the blast cell cytoplasm

A 26-year-old man presented with a two day history of spontaneous nose bleeding. Examination was unremarkable apart from skin pallor. Results of investigations are shown in **70**.

Questions
a What is the diagnosis?
b What further confirmatory tests would you do?

Data interpretation 18

The pedigree of a family with severe haemophilia A is shown in **71**. The alleles for each family member are for the intragenic factor VIII BclI polymorphic site (alleles 1.2 and 0.9 kb). The additional alleles for III$_7$–III$_{10}$ are for probe C, which detects an additional intragenic polymorphic BglI site (alleles 20 and 5 kb).

Questions

a Which individuals are obligate carriers?

b Could II$_3$ have haemophilia?

c On the basis of the BclI data is female III$_9$ a carrier?

d The individuals III$_7$–III$_{10}$ were reinvestigated using probe C. Can the carrier status of III$_9$ and III$_{10}$ be determined?

e Is fetus IV$_3$ affected by haemophilia?

f Explain how III$_2$ has alleles 1.2 and 0.9.

71

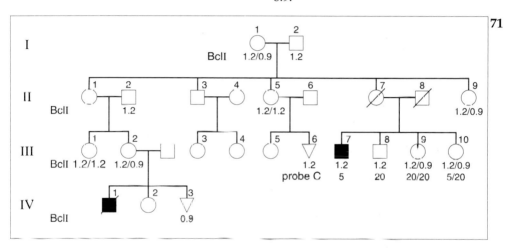

Data interprotation 19

A 28-year-old woman incurred a deep left thigh wound during a domestic dispute with her husband. FBC showed:
- Hb 8.4 g/dl;
- WCC 5.4 × 10^9/l;
- platelets 187 × 10^9/l.

The gash was sutured and the patient transfused four units of packed cells. She made a satisfactory recovery, but eight days after the first transfusion reported spontaneous bruising. Results of a coagulation screen and repeat FBC are shown in **72**.

72

Test	Result	Control
One-stage PT	18 secs	15 secs
KCCT	40 secs	44 secs
Hb	12.6 g/dl	
WCC	4.7 × 10^9/l	
Platelets	18 × 10^9/l	

Questions

a What is the likely diagnosis?

b What treatment options are available?

Data interpretation 20

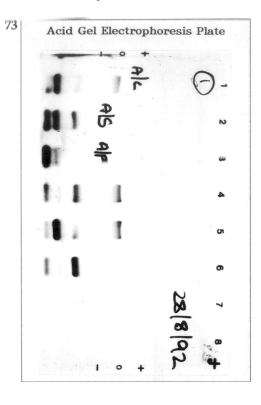

73

Acid Gel Electrophoresis Plate

A 58-year-old West Indian man was discovered to have a macrocytic mild anaemia as an incidental finding on a routine blood count. He required a very minor surgical procedure. He was fit and well and had no past medical history. The blood count revealed:
- Hb 12.4 g/dl (MCV 115.4 fl);
- RBC 3.24 × 10^{12}/l.

The peripheral film showed macrocytic red cells with many target cells and post-splenectomy changes. The acid gel Hb electrophoresis plate is shown (73). This patient's specimen has been run in lane 6.

Questions
a What is the diagnosis?
b Explain his lack of symptoms?
c What is the diagnosis of the patient whose specimen is in lane 4?
d What morphological features would be expected?

Data interpretation 21

74

Test	Result
Hb	9.2 g/dl
WCC	38 x 10^9/l
Atypical lymphocytes	30x10^9/l
Platelets	80 x 10^9/l
Blood film	Atypical lymphocytes, many having a multilobed nucleus
Immuno-phenotype	Strong positivity for CD2, CD3, CD4, CD5, and CD25 with HLA DR positivity; CD8 negative

A 40-year-old woman of West Indian origin presented with a spontaneous fracture of the upper third of her left humerus. She had been nonspecifically unwell for several months and had noticed a skin rash over her abdomen and trunk. Examination revealed shotty generalised lymphadenopathy with moderate hepatosplenomegaly and a discrete, raised, rose-coloured skin infiltrate over her upper chest and back. Results of tests are shown in 74.

Questions
a What is the diagnosis?
b What is the bone fracture due to?
c What investigation would confirm the diagnosis?

Data interpretation 22

Questions

a–j Which haematological diseases are associated with the cytogenetic abnormalities listed in 75?

Cytogenetic abnormalities associated with haematological diseases 75

a t(8;22)(q24;q11)

b Trisomy 12

c t(11;14)(p13;q11)

d inv(16)(p13;q22)

e Trisomy 8

f t(14;18)(q32;q21)

g t(2;8)(p12;p24)

h t(8;21)(q22;q22)

i 20q–

j High frequency of chromosomal and chromatid gaps, breaks, and rearrangements after exposure to mitomycin

Data interpretation 23

A 37-year-old woman presented with a vague history of tiredness for more than two years. Examination showed massive splenomegaly and a raised papular skin rash over the trunk and abdomen. Results of investigations are shown in 76.

Questions

a What is the diagnosis?

b How can this be distinguished from other lymphoid neoplasms?

c What is the prognosis?

Test	Result	76
Hb	10.4 g/dl	
WCC	$110 \times 10^9/l$	
Atypical lymphocytes	$96 \times 10^9/l$	
Platelets	$95 \times 10^9/l$	
Blood film	Mature lymphocytes with a folded nucleus; cytoplasm containing azurophilic granules	
Immuno-phenotype	CD1–, CD3+, CD4 , CD5–, CD8+, CD11+	
Cytogenetics	t(14;14)(q11;q32) in all cells examined	

Data interpretation 24

77

Test	Result
Hb	8.2 g/dl
WCC	4.6 x 10⁹/l
Neutrophils	0.6 x 10⁹/l
Atypical lymphocytes	3.0 x 10⁹/l
Platelets	61 x 10⁹/l
Bone marrow aspirate	Infiltration with 22% atypical lymphocytes, lymphocytes contained an eccentrically placed nucleus with fine chromatin condensation with pale slate-blue cytoplasm
Immuno-phenotype	CD11c+, CD22+, CD5–, CD8–, CD4–, CD25+
Cytogenetics	t(8;14)(q24;q32)
Cytochemistry Myeloperoxidase	Negative
PAS	Negative
Acid phosphatase	Generalised cytoplasmic positivity

A 44-year-old man presented with a two year history of recurrent minor infections. Examination revealed a fit-looking man with a spleen 10 cm below the left costal margin. There were no other clinical findings. Results of investigations are given in 77.

Questions

a What is the most likely diagnosis?
b Which features support it?
c How would you confirm it?

Data interpretation 25

A 12-year-old boy received an allogeneic bone marrow transplant for relapsed ALL. Two months after the transplant he developed a macular skin rash, and later dry mouth and eyes, buccal ulceration, and liver dysfunction. Six months post-transplant, he developed dyspnoea.

On examination he had bilateral wheezes and fine crackles. There was no preceding history of asthma. A chest radiograph showed air trapping.

Respiratory function tests showed an obstructive pattern. There was no benefit from bronchodilators.

Questions

a What is the differential diagnosis?
b What further investigations are necessary?

Data interpretation 26

A 4-year-old Caucasian girl has a history of jaundice associated with colds and other viral infections. When seen in clinic, investigations showed the results shown in **78**.

The osmotic fragility curve is shown (**79**).

Questions
a What is the diagnosis?
b How should this child be managed?

78

Test	Result	Normal
Hb	10.1 g/dl	
MCV	74 fl	
WCC	8.7 x 10^9/l (normal differential)	
Platelets	488 x 10^9/l	
Reticulocytes	15%	
DAT	Negative	
Hapto-globulin	<0.38 g/l	0.5–2.0
Pyruvate kinase	295 mu/10^9 RBCs	70–470 mu/10^9 RBCs
Acidified glycerol lysis time AGLT$_{50}$	6 mins 20 secs	> 30 mins

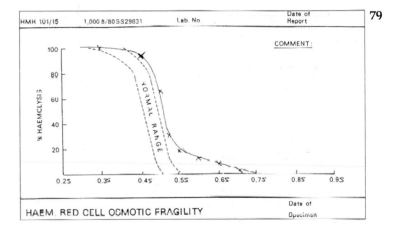

HMH 101/15   1,000 8/80 SS29831   Lab. No   Date of Report   79

COMMENT:

% HAEMOLYSIS

NORMAL RANGE

0.2S   0.3S   0.4S   0.5S   0.6S   0.7S   0.8S   0.9S

HAEM. RED CELL OSMOTIC FRAGILITY   Date of Specimen

Data interpretation 27

80

Test	Result	Normal
APTT	35 secs	28–38
PT	14 secs	13–16
Fibrinogen	1.7 g/l	1.5–4.0
Bleeding time template	11 mins	Up to 8
Platelets	250 x 10^9/l	
Factor VIII C	0.6 iu/ml	0.50–1.5
vWF antigen	0.82 iu/ml	0.45–1.40
vWF ristocetin co-factor	0.74 iu/ml	0.45–1.35

Platelet aggregation

Adrenaline	Primary aggregation only	
ADP	Primary aggregation only	
Collagen	Markedly reduced response	
Platelet ADP	3.5 mmol/ 10^8 platelets	2.5–6.0
Platelet ATP	4.2 mmol/ 10^8 platelets	3.3–8.0

5HT release

With ADP	2%	20–50%
Collagen	3%	25–50%

A 5-year-old boy has frequent spontaneous bruises and epistaxis. He requires tonsillectomy. Available information is shown in **80**.

Questions

a What is the diagnosis?

b What haemostatic therapy should be received before tonsillectomy?

Data interpretation 28

A 35-year-old woman presented with a two day history of blurred vision. Examination revealed generalised skin petechiae and a spleen which was just palpable. The fundi showed multiple small fundal haemorrhages and early papilloedema. Results of investigations are given in **81**.

Questions

a What is the diagnosis?

b Which features are characteristic of this disorder?

Test	Result	81
Hb	10.6 g/dl	
WCC	26 x 10^9/l (neutrophils 1.1 x 10^9/l, lymphocytes 2.7 x 10^9/l, blasts 20.6 x 10^9/l)	
Platelets	14 x 10^9/l	
Bone marrow	Almost entirely replaced with blasts similar to those seen in the blood film	
Cerebrospinal fluid	Mainly contains normal looking lymphocytes, but there is a small proportion of immature cells similar to those seen in the blood and marrow	
Cytogenetic studies	All cells examined showed a translocation t(9;11)(p22;q23)	
Cytochemistry of bone marrow		
Myeloperoxidase	Negative	
PAS	Mainly negative, but occasional cells showing fine positivity	
Naphthol AS acetate esterase (NASA)	Strongly positive (this reaction was inhibited by sodium fluoride)	
Acid phosphatase	Strongly positive with a diffuse and granular pattern	

Data interpretation 29

82

Test	Result	Normal
APTT	47 secs	28–38
APTT mix (50% patient; 50% normal incubated for 1 hour	45 secs	
PT	14 secs	13–16
Platelets	250 × 10⁹/l	
Factor VIII	0.60 iu/ml	0.50–1.5
Bleeding time	7 mins	Up to 8
Dilute Russell Viper venom time	Patient: control ratio 1.22	0.9–1.09
Correction test with platelet extract	Patient: control ratio 1.06	

A 46 year old lady said that she thought her grandfather had a bleeding disorder. She requires a hysterectomy for menorrhagia. Available information is shown in **82**.

Questions
a What is the cause of the abnormalities shown?
b What further investigations are indicated?
c Are any special precautions required at hysterectomy?

Data interpretation 30

83

Immunophenotype	Child a	b	c	d
CD2	2%	2%	60%	2%
CD7	2%	2%	70%	30%
CD10	5%	90%	2%	2%
CD19	80%	80%	2%	2%
CD13	3%	5%		60%
CD33				60%
CD34	75%			
CD45				70%
Tdt	70%		60%	
Cyt IgM		90%		
Surface IgM		1%		

Questions
a–d Discuss the significance of the immunophenotypes shown in **83** in childhood cancer.

Data interpretation 31

A 76-year-old man, who had been non-specifically unwell for 18 months, presented with a two week history of skin bruising and sore gums. Examination showed skin pallor, widespread petechiae, and mouth ulcers. Results of investigations are shown in **84**.

Questions
a What is the diagnosis?
b Describe the cytogenetic changes that can occur in this condition.

84

Test	Result
Hb	6.2 g/dl
WCC	21×10^9/l (neutrophils 0.2×10^9/l, blasts 9.1×10^9/l)
Platelets	5×10^9/l
Bone marrow	65% infiltration with small immature-looking myeloblasts; 15% abnormal erythroblasts, some with bilobed nuclei and megaloblastic changes
Cytochemistry (marrow cells)	
Myeloperoxidase	Positive
PAS	Negative
Cytogenetics	t (1;3) (p36;q21)

Data interpretation: answers

Data interpretation 1

a The diagnosis is von Willebrand's disease (vWD) and because the history is lifelong it is probably congenital. As the ristocetin co-factor activity is very much less than the factor VIIIC and vWF antigen concentration, the patient has type II vWD. This type contains a number of subtypes, which are classified by examination of the vWF multimeric structure.

b In the treatment of vWD it is best to try and avoid the use of blood products. However, in type II vWD, because of the functional deficiency of the vWF molecule, raising its concentration with DDAVP may not be sufficient to secure normal haemostasis. This can be assessed by a test dose of DDAVP and collection of sequential samples to measure vWF ristocetin co-factor response. If the maximum vWF ristocetin co-factor level, which usually occurs at 30–60 minutes, is less than about 0.20 iu/ml the response is inadequate to allow tooth extraction. It may be necessary to use a factor VIII concentrate. The vWF quality and quantity varies considerably between concentrates from different manufacturers. A concentrate should be chosen in which the vWF activity and multimeric structure is well preserved and in particular contains high molecular weight multimers. A single infusion immediately before surgery should be given along with tranexamic acid and an antibiotic, both of which should be continued for 10 days.

Data interpretation 2

a t(4;11) occurs in 2% of childhood ALL, and is associated with infant leukaemia, hyperleukocytosis, CD10 negative/CD19 positive (early pre B or null cell) ALL, myeloid antigen co-expression, and poor prognosis.

b t(1;19) occurs in 5% of childhood ALL, and is associated with CD10 positive/cytoplasmic immunoglobulin positive (pre-B) ALL. Although associated with a poorer prognosis in some studies, this remains unproven, and recent intensive protocols have not supported a difference in outcome compared with common ALL.

c t(8;14) is one of three translocations specifically associated with mature B cell (surface immunoglobulin positive) ALL/lymphoma. The breakpoint in chromosome 8 involves the c-MYC oncogene. Mature B cell ALL has had an extremely poor prognosis, but new intensive treatment protocols are associated with a high remission rate and probable long-term survival. B cell lymphoma in childhood is associated with abdominal bulk disease, and marrow and CNS involvement.

d Monosomy 7 has been associated with acute myeloid leukaemia, myelodysplasia and a myeloproliferative disorder of infancy with similar features, but different natural history to juvenile CML. Monosomy 7 is often a feature of secondary AML and myelodysplasia, and is associated with a poor prognosis.

e t(9;22) occurs in 2% of childhood ALL, and in children with the adult form of CML. In ALL, t(9; 22) is uniformly associated with a poor prognosis due to refractory disease or early treatment failure, and is a recognised indication for allogeneic bone marrow transplantation in first remission. The translocation breakpoint may differ between ALL and CML, with fusion gene products of different molecular weight (p190 and p210, respectively).

f t(8;21) is a characteristic finding in AML, and although most closely associated with FAB type M2, also occurs in other FAB types. It appears to be associated with a good prognosis, and the breakpoint on chromosome 21 involves the ETS oncogene.

Data interpretation 3

a Anti-e or occasionally anti-c.
b Anti-P.
c Anti-I.
d Anti-I.
e Anti-Pl^{A_1}.

f Anti-Gm. This is an antibody to the heavy chain of the IgG molecule, also known as RAGGS (rheumatoid agglutinators).
g Anti-i and also anti-I.

Data interpretation 4

a T cell acute lymphoblastic leukaemia (T-ALL).
b Expression of CD3 and CD7 are typical of T-ALL blasts. Other T cell markers (e.g. CD1, CD2, CD4, CD5, CD8) are heterogenously expressed.

c Age greater than 15 years; lymphadenopathy; high WCC at presentation. The expression of CD10 in T-ALL is associated with a better outcome.

Data interpretation 5

a Group O cord cells or adult group O patient with agammaglobulinaemia.
b Normal AB.
c Probable group O with autoantibody.
d Group A with acquired B. This may be seen in patients with carcinoma of the colon.

e Ax. A subgroup of A that gives a characteristic result of no agglutination with anti-A serum, 3+ with high titre serum.
f A2 with an anti-A1.

Data interpretation 6

a The automated differential count suggests a neutrophilia, but the neutrophil 'cloud' on the peroxidase channel is moved to the left and merges with the monocyte 'cloud'. This indicates myeloperoxidase (MPO) deficiency within the neutrophils. As a result the neutrophils are being identified as large cells with little endogenous peroxidase, as are monocytes. This will make it difficult for the automated cell counter to find a valley between the neutrophil and monocyte 'clouds' and may result in an inaccurate automated differential count. The peripheral blood morphology confirmed a neutrophilia with normal neutrophil morphological appearances.

b MPO deficiency is the most common inherited disorder of phagocytes. It is inherited in an autosomal recessive manner, the complete deficiency being seen in 1:4000 individuals and partial deficiencies in 1:2000. MPO catalyses the formation of hypochlorous acid from chloride and hydrogen peroxide in the neutrophil respiratory burst pathway. As a result there is a defect in *in vitro* killing of *Candida* spp. and *Aspergillus* spp. Despite this there is no increased incidence in infection in individuals with MPO deficiency except in those with concurrent diabetes mellitus in whom disseminated candidiasis may occur. In asymptomatic individuals no specific therapy is required.

Data interpretation 7

a Burkitt's lymphoma. This is a disease of B lymphoid cells with L3FAB morphology. In this patient, the case history and lymph node morphology are typical. The immunophenotyping pattern is that of a B cell lymphoma. The reciprocal translocation seen here is present in 80% of people with Burkitt's lymphoma.

b The disease is often multifocal at diagnosis. Staging investigations include CT scan of chest and abdomen. Bone marrow involvement is uncommon. Antibody to Epstein–Barr virus is usually positive.

Data interpretation 8

a The history is of an acute, warm haemolytic anaemia with IgG present on red cells, but no complement bound. Autoimmune haemolysis is often idiopathic in childhood, but may follow infection, or be associated with autoimmune disease, immune deficiency, or malignancy. The platelet count is normal, so there is no evidence of Evans' syndrome. The history of polyarthropathy and maternal nephritis are of concern, and screening for autoimmune disease is indicated. However, arthropathy may follow viral or streptococcal infection in children, and the ASO titre should be checked. There is a high reticulocyte count consistent with on-going haemolysis. A blood film should be examined, and would be expected to show polychromasia, and spherocytosis. Haematinics should be checked, as deficiency may precipitate exacerbation of anaemia. Other investigations would include renal function, and urine microscopy to exclude nephritis, and a study of antibody specificity.

b Management is by trial of steroids, and transfusion should be avoided, particularly as crossmatch may be difficult. If steroid response is adequate, these should be steadily tailed off to avoid steroid side-effects. If steroids fail, immunosuppression with azathioprine may help. Episodes of acute haemolysis may respond to intravenous immunoglobulin infusion. For children with severe, inadequately controlled haemolysis, splenectomy is effective in 50–70% of cases. Although best avoided in children under 6 years of age, this patient would be at lower risk of sepsis. Preparation before splenectomy includes vaccination against *Pneumococcus* and *Haemophilus*. Daily penicillin prophylaxis is essential until at least 18 years of age. Some authorities consider that it should be lifelong.

Data interpretation 9

a The most likely cause of the jaundice is hepatitis C. It is six weeks since the last blood transfusion and hepatitis C antibody formation can take four months to be detectable with currently available kits. An alternative diagnosis would be decompensated hepatitis B.

b The blood samples should be labelled 'high risk'.

Data Interpretation 10

At acid pH there is only one band visible in the A position, but at alkaline pH there is a fast band in addition to a band in the A position. The abnormal fast band was quantitated at 25% and was confirmed by the reference laboratory as HbJ. HbJ is due to single amino acid substitutions in the β chain, which alters its charge and hence mobility on electrophoresis. This Hb variant is usually of no clinical importance. Lane 2 demonstrates another fast band in addition to HbA and is HbI. Lane 4 demonstrates an abnormal band in addition to HbA running between the A and C positions. This is HbG.

Data interpretation 11

a The red cell mass is at the upper limit of normal for a male and the plasma volume is reduced. Consequently, the patient does have pseudo or stress polycythaemia with a reduced plasma volume and a normal red cell mass.

b The contributory factors to this condition are likely to be his alcohol intake, which causes a reduced plasma volume and may also suppress respiration. In addition, he is a heavy smoker, which may have caused his red cell mass to be at the upper limit of normal. Over 50% of patients with stress polycythaemia have red cell mass and plasma volume, which are within the normal range, but are at the upper and lower limits respectively. Current practice varies, but it is generally felt that these patients should be urged to reduce their alcohol and tobacco intake, as this may often lead to a correction of the haematological values. Should this not occur; venesection may be required to keep the haematocrit less than 0.50.

Data interpretation 12

a Acute myeloblastic transformation of chronic myeloid leukaemia.

b The i(17q) in Ph+ CML is exclusive to the blastic phase and appears to be associated with myeloid characteristics.

Data interpretation 13

a The results indicate that this lady is a carrier of haemophilia A. This diagnosis is based on the reduced factor VIIIC with normal vWF antigen and ristocetin co-factor levels. From these results it is not possible to know whether she is a carrier of mild, moderate or severe haemophilia.The alternative diagnosis is that she has a variant of von Willebrand's disease (vWD) in which there is a defect in the factor VIII binding site on vWF. This can be determined by nucleotide sequencing the relevant part of the vWF gene.

b By studying family members it might be ascertained whether any have laboratory characteristics of haemophilia A or vWD. Once correctly diagnosed the lady can be accurately counselled about the probability of having a child with a haemostatic disorder.

Data interpretation 14

a The investigations indicate aplastic anaemia, which can be classified as non-severe by the modified Camitta criteria. Severity is judged by the degree of pancytopenia and reticulocytopenia. Severe aplastic anaemia requires two out of three criteria (neutrophils less than $0.5 \times 10^9/l$, platelets less than $20 \times 10^9/l$, corrected reticulocyte count less than 1%). The elevated HbF is a feature of stress haemopoiesis. The normal cytogenetics after culture with DEB excludes Fanconi's anaemia, and the negative Ham's test excludes paroxysmal nocturnal haemoglobinuria (PNH), both of which may present as aplastic anaemia.

b Prognosis is related to the severity of neutropenia, and is particularly poor with neutrophils less than $0.2 \times 10^9/l$ (very severe aplasia).

c Management of aplastic anaemia in childhood is by allogeneic bone marrow transplantation if there is a matched family donor. Immunosuppression with ALG or cyclosporin may produce improvement, but long-term survival of children treated by immunosuppression is poor. Adult series indicate a high probability of clonal marrow disorders (AML, myelodysplasia, PNH) in survivors treated by immunosuppression.

Data interpretation 15

a B cell prolymphocytic leukaemia. Distinguishing features are massive splenomegaly without prominent lymphadenopathy, male sex, lymphocyte count higher than $100 \times 10^9/l$. The morphology is characteristically of large cells with prominent nucleoli, often with condensed chromatin. Cells show a B cell phenotype, but CD5 is often negative, an important distinction from B-CLL.

b Typically, six months to two years (i.e. a much more aggressive disease than B-CLL).

Data interpretation 16

a This child is G6PD deficient.

b Electrophoretic analysis in view of his ethnic background would identify him as G6PD A variant deficient (G6PD A⁻).

c Generally haemolysis is less severe with the African variant A⁻ compared to Mediterranean variants. Nevertheless there is a risk of haemolysis. Drug-induced oxidative haemolysis is less severe in the A⁻ variant, but great care should be taken particularly if antimalarial drugs are required. Individuals with the G6PD A⁻ variant are more susceptible to acute haemolysis associated with infection (e.g. *Salmonella*, β-haemolytic streptococci, and coliforms), and this may be because G6PD-deficient red cells are unable to withstand hyperthermia.

Data interpretation 17

a Acute myeloid leukaemia (FAB M7). The features of this are:

● a sudden onset of pancytopenia in the absence of organomegaly;

● variable number of circulatory blasts, which may exhibit cytoplasmic budding;

● hypercellular marrow with increased reticulin;

● trilineage dysplasia with a predominance of abnormal megakaryocytes; CD41 (glycoprotein IIb/IIIa) is a megakaryocyte marker and the chromosomal translocation is rare, but is associated with abnormal thrombopoiesis.

b Further immunophenotyping with CD42 (glycoprotein Ib) and CD61 (glycoprotein IIIa) should confirm the diagnosis.

Data interpretation 18

a I, II_1, II_7, and III_2 are obligate carriers.

b Yes because his mother is an obligate carrier.

c III_7 and III_8 both have the 1.2 allele, but only III_7 is affected, mother (II_7) is homozygous 1.2/1.2. Therefore it is not possible to determine whether III_9 is a carrier.

d It is known from the pedigree that II_7 is an obligate carrier. The data demonstrates that, as the haemophilia gene is linked to allele 5, that mother must be 5/20 and father 20. Therefore III_9 is not a carrier and III_{10} is a carrier because she has an allele of 5 kb.

e No, because he does not have the allele linked to haemophilia in this pedigree (1.2).

f Mother (II_1) is an obligate carrier and therefore must be 1.2/1.2. Father (II_2) of III_1 is 1.2. As daughter (III_2) is 1.2/0.9, her apparent father II_2 is not her genetic father because he is 1.2 and her genetic father must have been 0.9. This is therefore a case of non-paternity of III_2.

Data interpretation 19

a The most likely diagnosis is post-transfusion purpura occurring in those who are negative for the Pl A1 platelet-specific antigen. Thrombocytopenia is commonly seen about a week after transfusion of red cells or platelets, there being an anamnestic response and stimulation of anti-Pl A1 antibody. The exact mechanism is unknown, but the patient's own Pl A1 negative platelets are also destroyed in this immune reaction.

b The treatment options are Pl A1 negative platelets or infusions of intravenous immunoglobulin used in a similar manner as for the treatment of ITP. Plasmapheresis may also be tried. Occasionally this condition may be seen in individuals who are Pl A1 positive when other platelet-specific antigen systems may be involved.

Data interpretation 20

a The results of Hb electrophoresis indicate sickle cell disease (HbS). This is unusual in an asymptomatic patient of his age.

b There is a prominent HbF band on electrophoresis (quantitated at 22%). The high level of HbF will modify the sickle cell anaemia. The inheritance of hereditary persistence of fetal haemoglobin (HPFH) is genetically determined and in Afro-Caribbeans is caused by a deletion of the β and δ loci. The distribution of HbF is pancellular as can be demonstrated by acid elution (Kleihauer) staining of red cells. The persistence of a high HbF level is the most likely cause for this individual's asymptomatic course.

c The patient has HbSC disease.

d Morphologically there are impressive numbers of target cells and only very rarely irreversibly sickled cells. Haemolysis is less severe in SC disease compared with SS disease, which results in a higher haematocrit. People with SC disease have a smaller MCV and a higher MCHC than those with SS disease. Sickling crises are less frequent in SC disease, but splenomegaly, eye disease, and avascular necrosis of the femoral head are more common than in SS disease.

Data interpretation 21

a Adult T cell leukaemia-lymphoma (ATLL). (Note the Caribbean origin of patient, typical 'flower-like' nuclear irregularities, and typical immuno-phenotyping pattern.)

b Osteolytic lesion in humerus. This is seen in relatively few cases, but hypercalcaemia is common and thought to be related to the release of cytokines by malignant cells (especially parathyroid-related protein, interleukin-I and tumour necrosis factor B).

c HTLV-1 positivity.

Data interpretation 22

a Burkitt's lymphoma or B cell ALL (L3).

b CLL.

c T-ALL.

d AML–M4.

e MDS.

f Follicular lymphoma.

g Burkitt's lymphoma or B cell ALL (L3).

h AML–M2.

i Myeloproliferative disease.

j Fanconi's anaemia.

Data interpretation 23

a T cell CLL (Western type).

b Clinical and blood findings in this female should suggest the diagnosis. Immunophenotype is characteristic; (CD5– should exclude classical B cell CLL; CD4–/CD8+ excludes adult T cell leukaemia lymphoma). Cytogenetic anomaly can also be seen in T cell lymphomas.

c 2–3 years.

Data interpretation 24

a Hairy cell leukaemia (HCL).

b History (isolated splenomegaly with recurrent infections); bone marrow morphology; immunophenotype (hairy cells may express a wide variety of antigens, but CD11c, CD22, and CD25 positivity are characteristic). No consistent karyotype is seen in HCL, but translocations involving 14q are frequent.

c Tartrate resistant acid phosphatase (TRAP) is demonstrated in hairy cells in all cases; distinctive cylindrical structures known as ribosome-lamella complexes are demonstrable on EM in about 50% of cases.

Data interpretation 25

a This patient developed acute (skin rash) then chronic (Sjögren's syndrome, liver dysfunction) GvHD following allogeneic BMT. Treatment for these complications is immunosuppression, usually with a combination of cyclosporin and prednisolone. The onset of clinical signs of obstructive airways disease, confirmed by an obstructive pattern on respiratory function testing, is of concern in the setting of chronic GvHD, and may reflect opportunist infection (often adenovirus) or may be idiopathic. In either case, obliterative bronchiolitis may result, with progressive deterioration in respiratory function despite immunosuppression, although occasional benefit has been seen with steroids.

b Further investigations should include viral serology, viral culture of pharyngeal secretions, bronchoscopy with lavage for opportunistic infection, and transbronchial biopsy for histology and microbiology.

Data interpretation 26

a The diagnosis is hereditary spherocytosis (HS), which is consistent with spherocytic red cells seen on peripheral blood morphology. She is anaemic with a reticulocytosis and negative DAT, but with active haemolysis as demonstrated by the reduced haptoglobins. The osmotic fragility curve identifies a population of spherocytes, which are more susceptible to lysis. The AGLT is also abnormal. The red cell enzyme PK is within the normal range. In a Caucasian child this would be the commonest red cell enzyme deficiency associated with haemolysis.

b Rarely, during childhood, patients with HS may require blood transfusion, particularly for aplastic crises, which may be related to parvovirus B19 infection. Due to increased marrow erythropoiesis, there is an increased folate demand and folic acid supplementation is therefore necessary. Anaemia and to a certain extent red cell survival can be improved by splenectomy, which should be delayed until at least 10 years of age. Polyvalent pneumococcal vaccination should be given before splenectomy and penicillin taken daily following splenectomy. As with any chronic haemolytic anaemia there is an increased risk of pigment gallstones and gallbladder disease.

Data interpretation 27

a This boy has a platelet disorder because the bleeding time is prolonged in the presence of a normal platelet count and vWF level. Only primary aggregation was observed with ADP and adrenaline and the response to collagen was poor. This can either be due to a reduction in the ADP content of dense granules or a defect in the release mechanism. In this instance the ADP content is normal, but the release reaction assessed by first loading the platelets with ^{14}C-5HT is markedly impaired. Thus he has a release, or aspirin-like, defect. Clearly these laboratory findings could be due to aspirin ingestion and it is important to ask the parents carefully about this possibility. As platelet tests are rather temperamental it is important to repeat the investigations on at least one further occasion before making a definitive diagnosis.

b A platelet transfusion should be given immediately before surgery. Tranexamic acid and an antibiotic should be given pre-operatively and continued for 10 days.

Data interpretation 28

a Acute monocytic leukaemia (FAB class M5).
b Acute monocytic leukaemia is characterised by a strong NASA, which is inhibited by NaF. Alpha-naphthyl butyrate esterase (ANBE) is probably a preferable substrate because of a greater degree of specificity and a stronger reaction in monocytoid cells.

t(9;11)(p22;q23) is the most common chromosomal translocation seen in M5 and about 65% of all 11q anomalies occur in patients with M5. CNS involvement in M5 is not uncommon and probably occurs in 10–15% of patients, although some series quote even higher figures.

Data interpretation 29

a A lupus anticoagulant is present as the APTT is prolonged and does not correct with normal plasma, and the DRVTT is prolonged and is shortened by platelet extract. Her other coagulation parameters are normal and there is no laboratory evidence to suggest she has a bleeding disorder.
b She should be investigated for an anticardiolipin antibody; if present this would indicate that she has an antiphospholipid antibody. As lupus anticoagulants are found in association with autoimmune disorders and collagen disorders she should be screened for anti-dsDNA and autoantibodies.
c Lupus anticoagulants are associated with a predisposition to thrombosis. In addition as she is over 40 years of age and is having a hysterectomy it would be prudent to consider her as being at high risk of developing a postoperative DVT. She should therefore be treated postoperatively with intravenous heparin in sufficient dose to give an APTT ratio of 1.5–2.0.

Data interpretation 30

a The immunophenotype indicates early pre-B (null cell) ALL. CD2 and CD7 (T cell markers) are negative, and CD19 positivity indicates a B lineage. CD13 is a myeloid antigen. CD34 (stem cell glycoprotein) although a feature of early undifferentiated clones, and associated with poor prognosis in AML, may be detected in ALL at different stages of differentiation, and does not have clear prognostic value. Early pre-B ALL is not an independent prognostic indicator after allowance for age and presenting WCC.

b The immunophenotype indicates pre-B (cytoplasmic immunoglobulin positive) ALL. This immunophenotype is detected in 15% of childhood ALL. Although associated with a poor prognosis in some studies, this has not been a uniform feature with intensive treatment protocols. There is a strong association between pre-B ALL and t(1;19) on cytogenetics.

c The immunophenotype indicates T cell (CD2 and CD7 positive) ALL. T cell disease accounts for 15% of childhood ALL, and is associated with a mediastinal mass in 40% of cases. Although considered a poor prognostic group in some series, T lineage loses prognostic significance after allowance for presenting WCC and sex are made.

d The immunophenotype indicates acute myeloid leukaemia. The lymphoid markers (CD2, CD10, CD19) are negative. CD7 positivity is a recognised feature of AML, is described in 15% of childhood cases, and may be a poor prognostic feature.

Data interpretation 31

a Acute myeloblastic leukaemia with preceding myelodysplastic syndrome (MDS). Preceding MDS is suggested by the history, partial blast cell infiltration of marrow, dyserythropoiesis, and cytogenetic findings.

b Cytogenetic changes that can occur are:
- chromosomal loss or gain (−5; −7; −17; −Y; +8; +21);
- deletions (commonest only) 5q , 7q ;
- translocations (commonest translocations only) (1;3) (p36;q21); (1;7) (p11;p11); (2;11) (p21;q23).

Grey cases: questions

Grey case 1 (Part 1)

A 37-year-old man presented with a 24-hour nose bleed and his relatives had noticed that he had become confused and forgetful. He also had a three week history of spontaneous bruising.

On examination there was a widespread petechial rash over his lower extremities, fresh bleeding in the mucous membranes of the mouth, and extensive bilateral fundal haemorrhages. Vital signs were normal and there were no other physical signs except for slight confusion about previous events. The results of a FBC and a marrow aspirate were as follows:

- Hb 6.0 g/dl;
- WCC 210 x 10^9/l (neutrophils 5%, lymphocytes 1%, blasts 92%);
- platelets 15 x 10^9/l;
- bone marrow aspirate completely replaced with primitive-looking agranular myeloblasts.

Questions a–c
a What is the diagnosis?
b What further investigations are essential?
c What treatment is needed?

Grey case 1 (Part 2)

Following leucopheresis (WCC 72 x 10^9/l) and platelet transfusion, the patient improved with little if any evidence of confusion. The coagulation screen was normal and cytotoxic chemotherapy (adriamycin 45 mg/m^2 for 2 days, and cytosine arabinoside 200 mg/m^2/day for 5 days) was given by intravenous infusion.

After two treatments with an interval of three weeks, the marrow aspirate showed 22% myeloblasts. Treatment then followed with high-dose cytosine arabinoside (3 g/m^2/day for 5 days) and amsacrine (120 mg/m^2/day for 5 days). A prolonged period of neutropenia followed.

The results of a further aspirate and a blood count on the 52nd day after presentation were as follows:

- Hb 10.1 g/dl;
- WCC 1.1 x 10^9/l (neutrophils 0.45%)
- platelets 45 x 10^9/l;
- bone marrow aspirate showed blast cells in a recovering marrow.

Twenty-four hours later, the patient developed a fever (temperature 38.6°C) associated with a dry cough and rigors. The chest radiograph was clear and blood cultures subsequently showed no bacterial growth. Intravenous broad spectrum antibiotics (azlocillin and gentamicin) were started immediately. By the next day the patient had deteriorated and showed signs of acute respiratory distress. A further chest radiograph showed bilateral uniform shadowing throughout all lung areas.

Questions d–f
d What is the differential diagnosis and which diagnosis is most likely?
e What additional investigations would you consider?
f What further treatment is indicated?

Grey case 2 (Part 1)

A 25-year-old woman was admitted with a swollen left calf. She had been taking an oral contraceptive pill containing 30 μg of oestrogen. There was no past, or family history of venous thromboembolism. A venogram demonstrated thrombosis up to the left iliac vein. The contraceptive pill was stopped. A coagulation screen was performed and found to be normal.

Treatment was started with intravenous heparin. Two days later a citrated blood sample was taken and the results shown in **85** obtained.

Test	Result	Normal	85
Antithrombin III activity	0.58 iu/ml	0.80–1.20	
Protein C activity	0.68 iu/ml	0.67–1.38	
Total protein S	66%	64–154	
Free protein S	57%	61–143	

Question a
a Interpret the results and offer possible explanations for the abnormalities.

Grey case 2 (Part 2)

After six days of intravenous heparin the patient was started on warfarin and stabilised to give a prothrombin ratio of 2.5 International Normalised Ratio (INR). After three months a further citrated blood sample gave the results shown in **86**.

Test	Result	Normal	86
Antithrombin III activity	0.59 iu/ml	0.80–1.20	
Protein C activity	0.52 iu/ml	0.67–1.38	
Total protein S	51%	64–154	
Free protein S	49%	61–143	

Questions b, c
b Interpret these results.
c How would you manage this patient now?

Grey case 2 (Part 3)

Results from a citrated blood sample taken two months after stopping warfarin are shown in **87**.

Test	Result	Normal	87
Antithrombin III activity	0.57 iu/ml	0.80–1.20	
Antithrombin III antigen	0.95 iu/ml	0.80–1.20	
Protein C activity	0.69 iu/ml	0.67–1.38	
Total protein S	70%	64–154	
Free protein S	65%	61–143	

Questions d, e
d Interpret these results.
e How would you manage this patient in future?

Grey case 3 (Part 1)

A 16-year-old girl was seen as an emergency with a two day history of vomiting and blood-stained diarrhoea. She also had a cramp-like lower abdominal pain, which she felt was similar to her normal menstrual discomfort. There had been no haematemesis and no melaena. She had returned from a week's holiday in Spain three days before and was taking no medication. There was no significant past medical history, but her sister had coeliac disease and her uncle, who lived in the same house, had also had diarrhoea recently.

The findings on examination were as follows:
- temperature 37.8°C;
- pulse 85 beats/min, sinus rhythm;
- blood pressure 120/80 mm Hg;
- cardiovascular system, chest, and nervous system, normal;
- diffuse lower abdominal tenderness with guarding, but no rebound.

Questions a–c
a What is your initial diagnosis?
b What investigations would you request?
c How would you manage this patient?

Grey case 3 (Part 2)

Three days later, the vomiting had improved, but the diarrhoea had not settled despite regular medication, and the patient remained pyrexial. Sigmoidoscopy showed evidence of colitis, and stool and blood cultures had been negative. A diagnosis of inflammatory bowel disease was therefore considered. At 5 p.m., the Haematology Laboratory telephoned the results of her FBC:

- Hb 10 g/dl;
- WCC 11 x 10^9/l;
- platelets 30 x 10^9/l.

Questions d, e
d What is the differential diagnosis?
e What further investigations are required?

Grey case 3 (Part 3)

The results of further investigations are given in 88 .

Questions f–h
f What is the diagnosis?
g What confirmatory tests may now be done?
h How would you treat this condition?

Test	Result	88
Sodium	127 mmol/l	
Potassium	4 mmol/l	
Urea	12.3 mmol/l	
Creatinine	217 µmol/l	
DIC screen	Normal	
Bone marrow aspirate	Normal	
Peripheral blood film	Thrombocytopenia and red cell fragments	

Grey case 4 (Part 1)

89

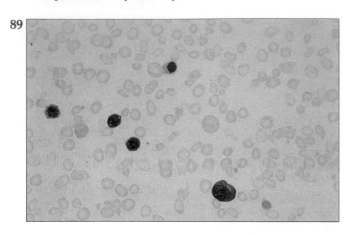

An Asian boy was seen at six months of age with:
- Hb 8.7g/dl (MCV 70 fl, MCH 22.8 pg);
- WCC 11.4 x 10⁹/l (normal differential count);
- platelets 310 x 10⁹/l.

A blood film is shown (89)

Questions a, b
a What is the probable diagnosis?

b What further investigations are needed?

Grey case 4 (Part 2)

This boy remained well achieving normal height and weight growth with Hb 8.9–9.9 g/dl during the next three years. At four years of age he was found to have 2 cm splenomegaly with frontal bossing and maxillary expansion. FBC results were:
- Hb 8.3 g/dl (MCV 63 fl);
- WCC 5.8 x 10⁹/l;
- platelets 300 x 10⁹/l;
- 3 nucleated RBCs/100 WBCs.

Questions c, d
c What clinical course is this boy demonstrating?

d Why may this occur?

Grey case 4 (Part 3)

At 5–6 years of age this patient's Hb began to fall, his splenomegaly increased to 6 cm, and he developed 5 cm hepatomegaly. In addition his height and weight fell from his previously well-maintained growth centiles and he became rather tired and listless. A chest radiograph revealed osteoporotic and enlarged ribs. FBC showed:
- Hb 5.0g/dl (MCV 68 fl, MCH 21.1 pg);
- WCC 5.2 x 10⁹/l;
- platelets 248 x 10⁹/l.

Questions e–g
e What clinical features are developing?

f What further investigations are required?

g How would you manage this patient?

Grey case 5 (Part 1)

A 22-year-old man with acute promyelocytic leukaemia (FAB M3) and a history of hepatitis B infection three years previously entered a stable remission and received a matched unrelated bone marrow transplant from a 45-year-old female donor.

Conditioning for the transplant was busulphan, 16 mg/kg, and cyclophosphamide 200 mg/kg, both drugs given in divided doses. Intravenous cyclosporin was used for post-graft immunosuppression, and the graft was T-cell depleted with a pan T cell monoclonal antibody. The patient received prophylactic septrin and colistin and was nursed in a laminar air flow unit. Because of fungal septicaemia during induction chemotherapy, he was given prophylactic oral fluconazole.

On day 8 after the transplant, the patient complained of diffuse upper abdominal pain and watery diarrhoea. On examination, his temperature was 38.6°C, pulse 95 beats/min and blood pressure 100/60 mm Hg. His skin was jaundiced, but otherwise appeared normal. Abdominal examination showed upper abdominal tenderness and the spleen tip could just be felt.

Questions a–c
a What is your differential diagnosis?
b How would you investigate this patient?
c How would you manage him?

Grey case 5 (Part 2)

Forty-eight hours later, the patient appeared pale and again complained of upper abdominal pain. He continued to have a temperature over 38°C and abdominal examination showed ascites with tenderness in the right upper quadrant. The liver edge could just be felt below the right costal margin. His jaundice now appeared more marked.
• Serum bilirubin 112 μmol/l.
• Alkaline phosphatase 235 iu/l.
• Aspartate transaminase 80 iu/l (normal range 0–45).
  FBC and blood film results were:
• Hb 8.0 g/dl;
• WCC 1 x 10^9/l;
• Platelets 8 x 10^9/l;
• Blood film showed occasional neutrophils (0.3x10^9/l) and occasional spherocytic red cells.

His diarrhoea was now very much less. There had been no clinical bleeding and occult blood tests on stool samples were negative.

Questions d–f
d What additional diagnoses should be considered?
e What further investigations are needed?
f What treatment changes would you make?

Grey case 5 (Part 3)

Questions g–i
g What is the cause of the abdominal signs and symptoms?

h How can this be confirmed?
i What factors may have predisposed to this diagnosis?

Grey case 6

90

Test	Result
Hb	3 g/dl
WCC	$3 \times 10^9/l$ (neutrophils 1, lymphocytes 1, blasts 0.5)
Platelets	$25 \times 10^9/l$
Bone marrow aspirate	Haemodilute, with occasional myeloid precursors and undifferentiated blasts
Bone marrow trephine	Myelofibrosis with islands of residual haemopoiesis, and prominent blasts
Marrow aspirate immuno-phenotype	
CD2	15%
CD5	27%
CD10	2%
CD13	14%
CD15	10%
CD19	8%
HLADR	22%
CD42	5%
Marrow cytogenetics	Showed the presence of a clone characterised by 48, XY, +21, +21

An 18-month-old boy with Down's syndrome was seen in Casualty with a five week history of pallor and bruising. On examination he had 4 cm hepato-splenomegaly. Results of investigations are shown in **90**.

Questions a, b

a Discuss the differential diagnosis.

b What haematological complications may occur in Down's syndrome?

Grey case 7 (Part 1)

A 50-year-old man of 70 kg is admitted with a large right thigh haematoma which developed over a five day period following a fall in his garden. Three years previously he bled for 12 hours intermittently after a molar tooth extraction. As a child he underwent tonsillectomy and circumcision without excess bleeding. He had one brother and two sisters; none had a history suggestive of a bleeding disorder.

On examination he had a large haematoma in his thigh with some superficial bruising visible. No other bruising was present. His large joints all appeared normal. The results of initial investigations are shown in **91**.

Questions a, b
a Discuss the abnormalities.
b What further investigations are appropriate?

91

Test	Result	Normal
Radiograph right thigh	No fracture	
Hb	10.3 g/dl	
WCC	9.3 x 10⁹/l	
Platelets	175 x 10⁹/l	
APTT	48 secs	28–38
APTT mix (50% patient, 50% normal) (incubated for 1 hour at 37°C)	44 secs	
PT	14 secs	13–16
Fibrinogen	3.2 g/l	1.5–4

Grey case 7 (Part 2)

Results of further tests are shown in **92**.

Questions c, d
c Interpret and comment on the results shown in **92**.
d How could the activity of inhibitors be further demonstrated and how should the patient be managed?

92

Test	Result	Normal
Factor VIIIC	0.11 iu/ml	0.50–1.50
vWF antigen	0.85 iu/ml	0.45–1.40
vWF ristocetin co-factor	0.72 iu/ml	0.45–1.35
Bethesda inhibitor assay	0.9 iu/ml	

Grey case 7 (Part 3)

The patient received 3000 units of human factor VIII concentrate.

Questions e, f
e Interpret the data shown in **93**.
f How should the patient be further managed?

93

Time	Factor VIIIC (iu/ml)
Pre-infusion	0.12
30 mins	0.32
60 mins	0.25
120 mins	0.20
180 mins	0.13

Grey case 8 (Part 1)

A 63-year-old man was admitted to the Medical Ward for investigation of 14 kg weight loss in the preceding three months. His appetite had been good, he had no night sweats, and he was otherwise uncomplaining. He was diagnosed as having diabetes mellitus nine years ago and this had later been controlled on diet and oral hypoglycaemics. He had had an episode of jaundice during the war while in Africa. Two of his brothers had died from gastrointestinal malignancy and he has one son and one daughter who are both alive and well.

On examination, he was thin with palmar erythema and bilateral Dupuytren's contractures. There was no clubbing. He did appear abnormally hirsute with scarring of the back of his hands and had 10 cm hepatomegaly, but no splenomegaly or ascites. There was some suggestion of a sensory peripheral neuropathy. Clinical examination was reported as otherwise normal.

Questions a, b
a What is your differential diagnosis?
b What investigations are indicated?

Grey case 8 (Part 2)

The results of the further investigations discussed in the answer to **b** are shown in **94**.

Question c
c What other investigation not listed would be most useful?

Grey case 8 (Part 3)

Questions d, e
d What is the diagnosis?
e What treatment is appropriate?

Grey case 8 (Part 4)

The patient continued to drink heavily. It was noted that there was:
• a steady increase in Hb to 18.7 g/dl;
• haematocrit 0.57;
• MCV 104 fl;
• WCC and platelets normal.

Questions f–h
f What is the likely diagnosis?
g What confirmatory tests can be done?
h What aetiological factors are important in this man?

Test	Result	Normal
Hb	15.9 g/dl	
MCV	105 fl	
WCC	Normal	
Platelets	Normal	
U&Es	Normal	
Alkaline phosphatase	120 iu/l	30–115 iu/l
Gamma GT	110 iu/l	0–45 iu/l
Chest radiograph	Obstructive airways disease; otherwise normal	
HbA$_1$	13%	5.7–8%
Blood glucose series		
6.00 a.m	16	
12.00 midday	12	
6.00 p.m	16	
Midnight	10	
Abdominal ultrasound	Homogeneous hepatomegaly. Normal spleen and kidneys	
Ferritin	2164 µg/l	15–300 µg/l
Urinary porphyrins	Normal	
Liver biopsy	Features of cirrhosis.Iron deposition in parenchyma, Kupffer cells, and portal tracts. No features of alcoholic hepatitis	

Grey case 8 (Part 5)

Six years after the initial diagnosis, this patient's liver function tests showed a marked deterioration as follows:
- alkaline phosphatase 495 iu/l;
- AST 275 iu/l (5–45 iu/l);
- bilirubin 38 µmol/l (0–17 µmol/l).

Depressed following the death of his wife six months earlier, he admitted drinking 1–2 glasses of wine daily. On examination, he was emaciated. He had palmar erythema, gynaecomastia, bilateral Dupuytren's contracture, 8–10 cm hepatomegaly, smooth, 3–4 cm splenomegaly, and no ascites.

Questions i, j

i What is the differential diagnosis?
j What further investigations are required?

Grey case 9 (Part 1)

A 9-week-old caucasian boy presented with rectal bleeding. Over the preceding few days he had been generally unwell with abdominal distension, poor feeding and listlessness. Two days before admission his mother had noticed blood in his stool and on the morning of admission she described a melaena stool. He had a rash on his face, which had been present for one day. There had been no antenatal problems and he was born by spontaneous vaginal delivery. His birth weight was 3.1 kg. There were no neonatal problems.

On examination he was pale and afebrile. He had bilateral occipital, axillary, and inguinal lymphadenopathy and a florid erythematous rash on his face, chest, and lower abdomen. His pulse rate was 110 bpm; cardiovascular and respiratory systems were normal. Examination of his abdomen revealed massive hepatomegaly (5 cm) and splenomegaly (12 cm).

Questions a, b
a What is the likely diagnosis?
b What initial investigations would you request?

Grey case 9 (Part 2)

95

Test	Result
Hb	6.6 g/dl
WCC	132 x 10^9/l (neutrophils 40%, lymphocytes 18%, monocytes 13%, eosinophils 8%, basophils 4%, blasts 12%, myelocytes 4%, promyelocytes 1%)
Platelets	17 x 10^9/l
Na$^+$	135 mmol/l
K$^+$	4.0 mmol/l
Urea	2.7 mmol/l
Creatinine	46 µmol/l
Phosphate	1.6 mmol/l
Bone marrow aspirate	Hypercellular, no megakaryocytes seen; micronormoblastic erythropoiesis; granulocytopoiesis shifted to the left with increased myelocytes, increased eosinophil precursors with cytoplasmic vacuolation; 1% myeloblasts
Cytogenetics	Normal

The results of initial investigations are are given in **95**.

Questions c, d
c What is the diagnosis?
d How would you manage this case?

Grey case 9 (Part 3)

Three months later this boy's blood count was:
- Hb 9.4 g/dl;
- WCC 13 x 10^9/l (neutrophils 53%, lymphocytes 24%, monocytes 16%, eosinophils 1%, basophils 2%, metamyelocytes 3%)
- platelets 261 x 10^9/l.

His hepatomegaly had completely resolved and spleen size had reduced to 5 cm. 6 mercaptopurine treatment was continued and stopped after 12 months. During the next two years the patient remained stable with FBC results in the region of:
- Hb 9.4–10.0 g/dl;
- WCC 8.4–10.6 x 10^9/l;
- platelets 226–451 x 10^9/l.

At three and a half years of age his mother complained that his abdomen was enlarging in size and despite being asymptomatic she was concerned about his abdomen. His Hb was 7.2 g/dl and he had a blood transfusion. One week later he was reviewed in clinic where he was well if pale, had 2 cm hepatomegaly, and 27 cm massive splenomegaly with dilated blood vessels over the chest wall. FBC results were:
- Hb 8.3 g/dl;
- WCC 9.3 x 10^9/l;
- platelets 144 x 10^9/l.

The peripheral blood film is shown (96).

Questions e, f

e What are the morphological features demonstrated in the blood film?

f What further investigations are required?

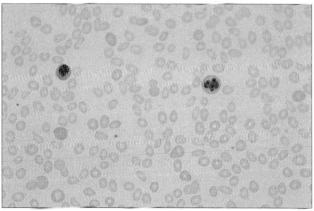

96

Grey case 9 (Part 4)

97

Test	Result
Differential WCC	
Neutrophils	33%
Lymphocytes	53%
Monocytes	5%
Eosinophils	2%
Basophils	1%
Cytogenetic studies	Normal

The results of these further investigations are shown in **97** and slides of the bone marrow trephine biopsy are shown in **98** (low power) and **99** (high power).

Questions g–i

g What important information is gained from the bone marrow examination?

h What is the underlying problem now affecting this child?

i How would you manage him?

98

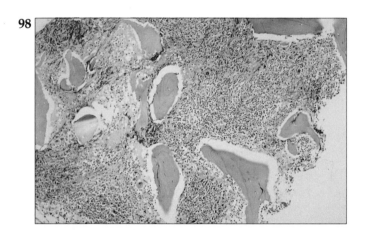

99

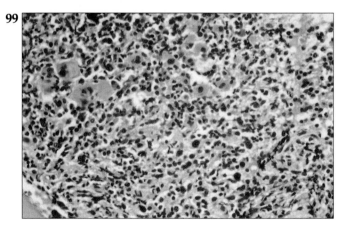

Grey case 10 (Part 1)

A 22-year-old man presented with a two week history of tiredness and bruising with nose bleeds on the two days before admission. He had no previous illnesses except conjunctivitis, which had been treated with eye drops on two separate occasions, six months and three months previously.

Examination confirmed skin pallor and showed multiple petechiae over the legs. Mucous membranes were normal, but both fundi showed several small retinal bleeds. Blood count showed:
- Hb 5.5 g/dl;
- WCC 2.6 x 10^9/l (neutrophils 0.4 x 10^9/l);
- platelets 17 x 10^9/l.

No abnormalities were seen on the blood film.

Questions a–e
a What is the most likely diagnosis?
b How would you confirm this?
c What eye drops did the patient probably have?
d How do they relate to the patient's blood disorder?
e What treatment would you advise?

Grey case 10 Part 2

Following a leucocyte-depleted blood transfusion, Hb increased to 10.6 g/dl. Three siblings were tissue-typed, but all mismatched. About a month after presentation, the patient was noted to be lightly jaundiced and complained of passing dark brown urine, especially noticeable at night.

Questions f–i
f What has caused these symptoms and signs?
g How would you prove this diagnosis?
h What treatment is required?
i What further measures should be considered for the severe aplasia?

Grey case 10 Part 3

The Ham's acidified serum lysis test was strongly positive and there was a partial response to prednisolone, which was used at a maintenance dose of 10 mg daily. A matched unrelated donor transplant was carried out, following cyclophosphamide and total body irradiation as conditioning, and using partial T-cell depletion of the graft. After grade III recurrent acute graft versus host disease, which was suppressed with high-dose methylprednisolone, the patient's blood count returned to normal. Four months post-transplant he was well and receiving only cyclosporin and ciprofloxacin.

Shortly afterwards he presented with a gradual onset of breathlessness. On examination, he was breathless on minimal effort with reduced air entry to all areas of his chest. A chest radiograph showed normal lung fields; pulmonary function tests showed markedly reduced carbon monoxide gas transfer. He also complained of inability to clench his fists and had patches of smooth tight-looking skin over the backs of his hands and elbows.

Questions j–l
j What is the cause of the lung defect?
k How should it be treated?
l What is the skin abnormality?

Grey case 11

100

Test	Result
Hb	6.4 g/dl
WCC	5 x 10^9/l (neutrophils 1.5 x 10^9/l, lymphocytes 1 x 10^9/l, monocytes 1.5 x 10^9/l, eosinophils 0.7 x 10^9/l, blasts 0.05 x 10^9/l, nrbc 0.2 x 10^9/l)
Platelets	115 x 10^9/l
Bone marrow aspirate	Hypercellular with myeloid hyperplasia, no increase in blasts and minor dysplastic changes in the myeloid series. Megakaryocytes increased
Marrow cyto-genetics	Normal
Liver function tests	Normal
Virology	Normal
Auto-antibody screen	Normal
Serum IgG IgM	1.6 g/dl (normal 3–13) 3.9 g/dl (normal 0.5–2)
Cell-mediated immunity	Normal

A 1-year-old boy was referred following three months of poor weight gain, abdominal swelling, and pallor. There was no significant past medical history, and he was the product of a normal term delivery. He was developmentally normal.

On examination he had an 8 cm spleen, 4 cm liver, and minor lymphadenopathy. There were no stigmata of liver disease. The results of investigations are shown in 100.

Questions a, b
a Discuss the differential diagnosis.
b Discuss further investigations of this child.

Grey case 12 (Part 1)

A 25-year-old woman feeling well at 36 weeks' gestation in her first pregnancy was found to have the FBC shown in **101**. No previous blood counts were available, and there was no history of excessive bruising or bleeding. Her blood pressure was 140/90 mm Hg.

Test	Result	101
Hb	10.7 g/dl	
WCC	7.9×10^9/l	
Platelets	70×10^9/l	
Film	Normal red cell and platelet morphology	

Questions a, b

a What are the most likely conditions causing the thrombocytopenia.

b What further investigations are required?

Grey case 12 (Part 2)

Marrow aspirate revealed a cellular sample with a normal number of megakaryocytes. Some degree of myeloid hyperplasia was noted, but erythroid activity was normal. Stainable iron was present, but reduced. The results of other tests are shown in **102**.

Test	Result	Normal	102
APTT	38 secs	28–38	
PT	15 secs	14–17	
Fibrinogen	1.6 g/l	1.5–4.0	
Bilirubin	10 µmol/l	2–17	
ALT	42 iu/l	10–40	
Alkaline phosphatase	103 iu/l	40–125	
Reticulocytes	1.8%		
U&Es	Normal		
Viral titres	No recent infection identified		
Autoantibodies	Negative		
Coomb's test	Negative		
Urate	0.27 mmol/l	0.12–0.36	
Urinary protein	<0.2 g/24 hours		

Questions c, d

c Discuss these data and reach a working diagnosis.

d Discuss the management you would recommend during the rest of her pregnancy.

Grey case 13 (Part 1)

A 7-year-old boy, the only child of healthy parents, was referred with a five day history of general malaise, lethargy and bruising. He had lost his appetite and had recently been treated by his general practitioner with antibiotics for a sore throat. His school teacher had witnessed a shivering episode in class and had asked for him to be collected from school. His mother brought him straight to hospital. He had been born at term with a birth weight of 2.2 kg and needed to spend some time on the special care baby unit because of poor feeding. He was noted to have a small head and undescended testes. Apart from an orchidopexy aged four years there was no past medical history.

On examination he was pale, thin and afebrile. He was microcephalic. There was a petechial rash over his shoulders. There were no other abnormalities. His FBC showed:

- Hb 2.4 g/dl;
- MCV 112 fl;
- WCC 1.1 x 10^9/l (neutrophils 55%, lymphocytes 40%, monocytes 5%);
- platelets 10 x 10^9/l.

Questions a, b

a What is the differential diagnosis?
b What further investigations are required?

Grey case 13 (Part 2)

103

Test	Result
Biochemistry	Normal
Bone marrow aspirate	Hypocellular; no megakaryocytes seen; reduced myelopoiesis; severely megaloblastic erythropoiesis; M:E ratio 1:3.5; non-erythroid cells comprised plasma cells, histiocytes, lymphocytes, and mast cells
Bone marrow trephine	Hypocellular; increased fat spaces with a few islands of residual erythroid and myeloid cells; prominent plasma cells (see 104)
Blood chromosomes	Normal, no chromosome breaks
Hb F	14%
Viral studies	
Hepatitis A	Negative
Hepatitis B	Negative
Parvovirus B19	Negative
Skeletal survey	Normal

The results of investigations are shown in 103.

Questions c, d

c What is the diagnosis?
d What management would you suggest?

104

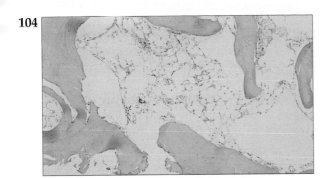

Grey case 13 (Part 3)

This boy was given a combination of ATG (horse), steroids, and cyclosporin A, which was uneventful. Four months later he had shown no response, requiring blood transfusions every 4–6 weeks and platelet transfusion for symptomatic bleeding/purpura. He was due to be admitted for a second course of ATG (rabbit), but became breathless and tachypnoeic with loss of appetite.

On examination there were blood blisters on his lips and tongue, his pulse was 120 bpm, blood pressure 110/80 mm Hg, and respiratory rate 40/min. There were no signs on auscultation and oxygen saturation was 77%. Chest radiograph was highly suggestive of *Pneumocystis carinii* pneumonia. He was treated with high-dose intravenous co-trimoxazole with steroids. There was a good initial improvement in his symptomatology, gases, and chest radiograph. Ten days into treatment he complained of pleuritic chest pain and developed two skin lesions, one on his leg (105) and one on his face (106).

105

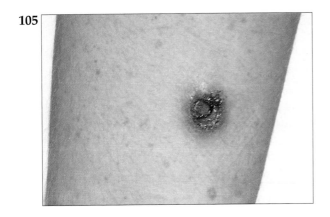

106

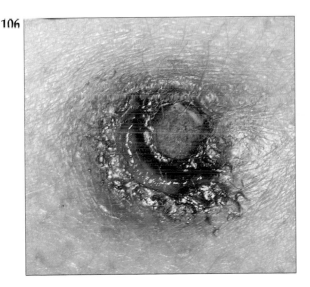

Questions e–g

e What is the most likely infecting organism?

f What is the most appropriate management?

g How do you perceive the management of this child's aplastic anaemia?

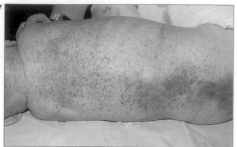

107

Grey case 14

An 11-month-old boy was referred with an extensive skin rash (**107**), and discharge from his ears. Examination showed generalised lymphadenopathy, and hepatosplenomegaly. FBC showed:
- Hb 7 g/dl, with normal red cell indices;
- WCC 12 x 10^9/l (neutrophils 9 x 10^9/l);
- platelets 120 x 10^9/l.

Questions a, b
a What is the likely diagnosis?
b What investigations are indicated?
c What is the management?
d What is the prognosis?

Grey case 15 (Part 1)

A 31-year-old woman attends the Antenatal Booking Clinic. She is 12 weeks pregnant. Her obstetric history is gravida 3 para 0. She received a transfusion of two units of blood 12 years ago following a major road traffic accident. Results of investigations were as follows:
- Hb 11.2 g/dl (MCV 94 fl);
- WCC 5.5 x 10^9/l;
- platelets 320 x 10^9/l;
- group and screen A Rh-negative; anti-D and anti-Kell present.

Questions a–c
a How do you explain the presence of the antibodies in the mother's serum?
b Is further testing indicated at this stage?
c How regularly would you see the mother during the pregnancy?

Grey case 15 (Part 2)

The mother is regularly reviewed during the pregnancy. Her anti-D levels are given in **108**.

Gestation (weeks)	anti-D (iu/ml)	108
12	2	
16	3	
20	3	
24	4	
28	6	

Question d
d At what stage is amniocentesis indicated?

Grey case 15 (Part 3)

The results of serial amniocentesis are shown in **109**.

Questions e, f
e Should induction of labour be considered?
f What further helpful result can amniocentesis provide which will assist your decision?

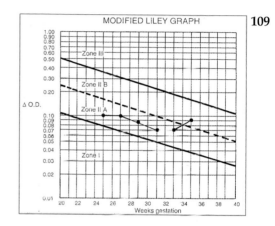

Grey case 15 (Part 4)

At birth:
- the baby is found to be A Rh-positive;
- direct Coomb's test was positive on cord cells;
- Hb 9.8 g/dl;
- bilirubin 120 μmol/l;
- red cell eluate reveals anti-D and anti-Kell;
- maternal screen reveals anti-D and anti-Kell.

Questions g i
g Should the baby receive any further treatment?
h Is the anti-Kell contributory to the haemolytic disease of the newborn?
i Should the mother receive prophylactic anti-D?

Grey case 16 (Part 1)

110

Test	Result
Hb	9.2 g/dl
MCV	84 fl
WCC	85x10^9/l (neutrophils 60%, lymphocytes 11%, monocytes 3%, metamyelocytes 10%, myelocytes 5%, basophils 1%, eosinophils 1%, nucleated red cells 4%)
Platelets	485 x 10^9/l
Blood film	Leucoerythroblastic anaemia, a number of macrocytes, and some misshapen red cells, including some tear drop forms. Several giant platelets
Bone marrow aspirate	Very cellular, reflecting the abnormalities seen in the blood film and also dyserythropoiesis with early megaloblastic changes. Normal megakaryocyte morphology

A 73-year-old woman presented with a six month history of weight loss and tiredness. For about six weeks, she had noticed aching pain in her left upper abdomen and examination showed splenomegaly which filled the whole abdomen. There were no other abnormal findings. The results of investigations are shown in 110.

Questions a, b
a What is the differential diagnosis?
b What further investigations are indicated?

Grey case 16 (Part 2)

111

Test	Result
Bone marrow trephine	Confirmed the proliferation of white cells, but showed an absence of reticulin
Karyotype	No chromosomal abnormality seen
BCR gene rearrangement	Showed a BCR-ABL protein of 210 Kd
Serum folic acid	2.4 µg/l (normal range 1.6–6.0 µg/l)
Serum vitamin B$_{12}$	126 ng/l (normal range 120–600 ng/l)

Results of further investigations shown in 111 suggest Philadelphia-negative, BCR-positive chronic myeloid leukaemia. Ph-negative CML occurs in about 5–10% of patients. About 33% have other cytogenetic anomalies, especially trisomy 8 and reciprocal translocations between chromosome 9 band q34 and a chromosome other than 22.

Treatment started with hydroxyurea 2.5 g/day. After 10 weeks the WCC was well controlled (5.6 x 10^9/l with normal differential), but platelet count had risen to 965 x 10^9/l. The spleen had reduced in size, but remained palpable approximately 12 cm below the ribs.

Question c
c What further treatment should be considered?

Grey case 16 (Part 3)

Alpha-interferon, 3 mega units three times weekly, was added and hydroxyurea continued at a maintenance dose of 1.0 g/day. After three weeks of outpatient treatment, the patient was admitted with a fever for 48 hours and severe pain in the centre of her chest for 12 hours. The pain was worsened by swallowing and associated with similar pain in the left shoulder. The left buccal mucous membrane was ulcerated and infected with *Candida*. Results of examination and investigations are as follows:

- temperature 37.8°C;
- pulse 110/min sinus rhythm;
- BP 140/85 mm Hg;
- Hb 9.8 g/dl;
- WCC $1.8 \times 10^9/1$ (neutrophils 40%, lymphocytes 60%);
- platelets $506 \times 10^9/1$.

Question d
d What is the differential diagnosis and what investigations should be done?

Grey case 17 (Part 1)

A 17-month-old boy was admitted with an eight day history of conjunctivitis, coryza, fever, and cough. There had been a suspicion of respiratory tract infection and he had been prescribed amoxycillin by the general practitioner. His parents had noted that he had become increasingly tired and irritable. Two days before admission he had a fever, a blood-stained nappy, and had become very pale. There was no significant past medical history.

On examination he was pale and drowsy. There was no lymphadenopathy, no rash, and mild jaundice.

Cardiovascular and respiratory systems were normal. Examination of the abdomen revealed a 1 cm enlarged liver. FBC showed:
- Hb 4.4 g/dl;
- MCV 80fl;
- WCC $25.3 \times 10^9/1$ (neutrophils 63%, lymphocytes 30%, monocytes 7%);
- platelets $438 \times 10^9/1$.

Questions a, b
a Look at the blood film (112). What are the morphological abnormalities?
b What further investigations are required?

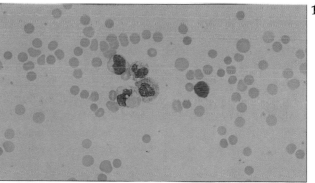

112

Grey case 17 (Part 2)

113

Test	Result
Bilirubin	79 µmol/l;
ALT	20 iu/l
ALP	444 iu/l
Albumin	39 g/l
Urate	0.5 mmol/l
Na^+	140 mmol/l
K^+	4.9 mmol/l
Urea	10.4 mmol/l
Creatinine	57 µmol/l
PT	17 secs (control 13 secs)
Thrombin time	11 secs (control 11 secs)
KCCT	34 secs (control 36 secs)
Direct antiglobulin test	Broad spectrum visual positive, anti-IgG negative, anti-IgA negative, anti-IgM negative, anti-C3 visual positive
Reticulocytes	3.5%
Blood cultures	No growth
Virology titres	No positive titres; parvovirus B19 negative
Mycoplasma titre	Negative
Immuno-globulins	Normal

The results of further investigations are shown in **113**.

Questions c, d
c What is the diagnosis and how would you confirm it?
d How would you manage the patient?

Grey case 18 (Part 1)

A 21-year-old woman, having had an uneventful first pregnancy, gave birth to a baby who developed jaundice in the first 24 hours of life. Antenatal testing of the mother at 12 and 34 weeks of the pregnancy revealed her to be O Rh-positive with a negative antibody screen. The mother took no medication throughout the pregnancy. During her adolescence, she suffered from skin rashes, arthralgia, and patchy hair loss, which was never fully investigated.

Questions a, b
a What further testing is required?
b Should the mother be given prophylactic anti-D?

Grey case 18 (Part 2)

Twelve hours after birth, the baby is noted to be bleeding from a venepuncture site. A coagulation screen is ordered which revealed:
- PT 19/14;
- KCCT 48/41.

Question c
c What are the possible diagnoses?

Grey case 18 (Part 3)

Investigation of the mother revealed:
- Hb 10.8 g/dl;
- WCC 9.8 x 10^9/l;
- platelets 243 x 10^9/l;
- antinuclear factor negative.

Questions d–f
d What is the likely diagnosis?
e What further tests are required?
f What treatment can be given to the baby?

Grey case 19

A 12-year-old girl was referred with lethargy, nausea and skin rash. She had been treated with 2 weeks Co-trimoxazole and iron sulphate tablets. Two months previously she had been on holiday in Malta.

On examination she was an ill girl, with no fever, but rigors. Examination revealed 10-cm splenomegaly.

Full blood count showed Hb 9.7 g/dl, WBC 2.5 (neutrophils 1) and platelets 137 x 10^9/l. A bone marrow aspirate and trephine were performed, and a slide of the aspirate is shown (114).

Questions a, b
a What investigations are indicated?
b Comment on diagnosis and treatment

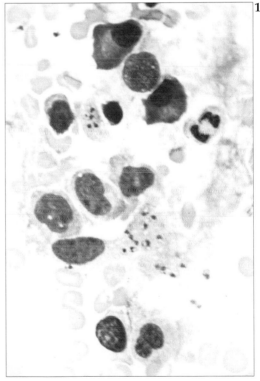
114

93

Grey case 20 (Part 1)

115

Test	Result	Normal
Hb	10.9 g/dl	
WCC	12.3 x 10⁹/l	
Platelets	25 x 10⁹/l	
APTT	39 secs	28–38
PT	16 secs	13–16
Fibrinogen	1.6 g/dl	1.5–4.0

A 65-year-old woman underwent uneventful cholecystectomy; she received heparin 5000 units b.d. as DVT prophylaxis. On admission and at three days post operation her blood counts had been normal. Mobilisation and discharge from hospital were delayed by a wound infection.

On the 11th post-operative day she developed colicky abdominal pain. Her right calf had become a little uncomfortable.

On examination she was pyrexial 38°C, pulse 90/min, chest clinically clear. Her abdomen was generally tender with some guarding; bowel sounds were very infrequent. The following results immediately available are shown in **115**.

Questions a, b
a Give a differential diagnosis.
b Suggest further investigations.

Grey case 20 (Part 2)

The venogram revealed thrombus extending from the right calf to the IVC. Plain abdominal radiographs did not reveal any fluid levels. A chest radiograph was normal. Whilst these investigations were being gathered the patient's condition deteriorated. The abdominal pain worsened and she had some melaena. Her pulse increased to 120/min and BP fell to 110/60 mm Hg.

At laparotomy, mesenteric artery thrombosis was found and a segment of ischaemic small bowel was excised.

Questions c, d
c What is the most likely haematological diagnosis?
d What management would be appropriate?

Grey case 21 (Part 1)

A 23-year-old woman presented with a short history of recurrent fever and weight loss of approximately 5 kg. She also complained of aching pains in small joints. Examination confirmed a fever of 37.8°C and showed discrete, raised, reddish lumps, about 1 cm in diameter, over the front of both legs below the knee. Other examination was negative except for splenic enlargement 2 cm below the left rib margin. The results of investigations are shown in **116**.

Test	Result	116
Chest radiograph	Symmetrical bilateral hilar enlargement	
Radiographs of hands, wrists and ankle joints	Unremarkable	
Hb	10.6 g/dl	
WCC	$10.1 \times 10^9/l$ (normal differential count)	
Platelets	$165 \times 10^9/l$	
Blood film	Normal	

Questions a, b

a What is the most likely diagnosis?
b What further investigations would you advise?

Grey case 21 (Part 2)

Over the next month, the patient lost a further 5 kg in weight and complained of excessive sweating, especially at night. She also noticed pain in her back after drinking alcohol.

Questions c–e

c What additional diagnosis should now be considered?
d What further investigation should be considered?
e How would you confirm the diagnosis?

Grey case 21 (Part 3)

Questions (f, g)

f What histological subtype of disease is most likely?
g How would you treat this patient?

Grey case 22

117

Test	Result	Normal
Hb	7.8 g/dl	
MCV	84 fl	
WCC	13.4 x 10⁹/l (neutrophils 2.8 x 10⁹/l)	
Platelets	21 x 10⁹/l	
Film	Fragmented red cells	
PT	25 secs	13–17
APTT	76 secs	26–35
Thrombin time	19 secs	10–12
Fibrinogen	1.1 g/l	1.5–4.0
AST	646 iu/l	10–40
Bilirubin	133 µmol/l	1–17
Albumin	29 g/l	
Triglycerides	Elevated	

An Asian boy, the first child of a first cousin marriage was admitted at eight weeks of age with a one week history of intermittent diarrhoea and a three day history of fever, breathing difficulties, and abdominal distension.

On examination he had widespread petechiae, tachypnoea, and massive hepatosplenomegaly. Chest radiograph showed cardiomegaly, small bilateral pleural effusions, and pulmonary infiltrates. Results of a FBC and other tests are shown in 117.

The child's condition deteriorated, and he was admitted to intensive care, intubated, and ventilated. His disseminated intravascular coagulation (DIC) was managed with blood product support and he was started on broad-spectrum antibiotics in view of his fever. However urine, sputum, and blood cultures had no growth. A bone marrow aspirate (118) and CSF cytospin (119) were performed.

Questions a–c
a What features are demonstrated in the bone marrow and CSF?
b What is the diagnosis?
c What is the management of this condition?

118
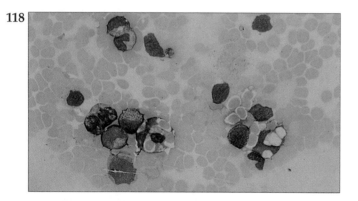

119
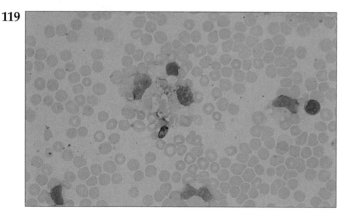

Grey case 23 (Part 1)

A 50-year-old man was seen in the Out-patient Department with a three month history of fatigue, light-headedness, and occipital headaches. He reported that after 20 minutes' walking, he needed to rest because of fatigue and stiffness in his thighs and shins. He suffered mild shortness of breath on exertion, but there was no paroxysmal nocturnal dyspnoea or orthopnoea and no chest pain. His appetite had been poor for a year, but his weight had remained steady and he had no night sweats. In the past he had undergone cataract extraction three years previously, which was uneventful. He is currently taking no medication. He came originally from Pakistan, but had lived in the UK for the past 15 years. He works as an accountant, smokes 15 cigarettes a day, and drinks alcohol only occasionally.

Physical examination was unremarkable, apart from a palpable splenic tip. The results of initial investigations were as follows:

- urea and electrolytes normal;
- liver function tests normal apart from a bilirubin of 84 µmol/l (0–17 µmol/l);
- ESR 150 mm/hr.

His FBC showed:

- Hb 5.9 g/dl (MCV 108 fl);
- WCC 5.8×10^9/l;
- platelets 340×10^9/l.

Question a

a What further investigations are required?

Grey case 23 (Part 2)

The results of further investigations are shown in **120**.

Questions b, c

b What is the likely diagnosis?
c What is the management?

Grey case 23 (Part 3)

Two days later, his Hb was 4.8 g/dl, and the patient was symptomatic as a result of his anaemia.

Question d

d Is blood transfusion indicated?

120

Test	Result	Normal
Serum B$_{12}$ and folate	Normal	
Reticulocytes	99×10^9/l	20–90
Direct Coomb's test	3+ positive for IgG and complement	
Autoantibody screen	Negative	
Serum electrophoresis	Normal	
Film	Macrocytes, nucleated red blood cells, tear drops, and spherocytes	
Bone marrow	Erythroid hyperplasia with megaloblastic changes	

Grey case 23 (Part 4)

The patient was successfully transfused four units of packed cells. Over the next month, steroids were decreased to prednisolone 15 mg daily. At that time, his Hb was maintained at around 10 g/dl. Subsequent investigations in an attempt to elucidate the cause of the autoimmune haemolytic anaemia included a chest radiograph, which was reported as normal, and CT scan of the abdomen, which showed slight splenomegaly.

One month later, there was a further episode of haemolysis and the prednisolone was increased to 30 mg daily. In addition, azathioprine, 50 mg t.d.s. was prescribed. Two weeks later, his Hb was 6 g/dl. At this time, a repeat bone marrow showed erythroid hypoplasia.

Questions e–g

e What may have happened?
f What diagnoses should be considered?
g What is the further management?

Grey case 23 (Part 5)

Three months after presentation, it was decided that the patient should be submitted for splenectomy.

Question h

h What prophylactic measures need to be taken in such patients?

Grey case 23 (Part 6)

The patient made a good recovery from splenectomy, but it proved to be an ineffective measure and the Hb remained low. A repeat bone marrow one month after stopping the azathioprine once again showed pure red cell aplasia.

Questions i, j

i What diagnosis must be considered now?
j What further therapeutic measures may be effective?

Grey case 24 (Part 1)

A 76-year-old woman, who had been previously well, presented with a sudden onset of severe shoulder tip pain made worse by deep inspiration or coughing. Examination showed a spleen enlarged 6 cms below the left ribs and a liver which was just palpable. Several small shotty lymph nodes were palpable in the neck and in both axillae. The results of a full blood count are shown in **121**.

Test	Result	121
Hb	9.6 g/dl	
WCC	36 x 10⁹/l (neutrophils 68%, monocytes 4%, lymphocytes 8%, metamyelocytes 14%, myelocytes 1%, eosinophils 1%, basophils 3%, nucleated red blood cells 1%)	
Platelets	96 x 10⁹/l	
Blood film	Red cells showed marked anisocytosis and poikilocytosis with occasional tear drop cells	

Questions a–e
a What is the most likely diagnosis?
b What is the cause of the patient's pain?
c What additional diagnosis should be considered?
d What additional physical sign might you associate with the enlarged spleen?
e What further investigation would you do to establish the diagnosis?

Grey case 24 (Part 2)

Further information is as follows.
• A karyotype on bone marrow cells showed a complete translocation between chromosomes 3, 11, and 13, present in 3 of 20 cells examined. The karyotype was otherwise normal.
• Molecular genetic studies for the BCR gene rearrangement showed a 210 kd BCR-ABL protein.

• Bone marrow aspirate and trephine showed a very cellular marrow reflecting the changes seen in the blood and with almost complete absence of reticulin.

Questions f, g
f What is the diagnosis?
g What treatment would you advise?

Grey case 24 (Part 3)

122

Test	Result
Hb	11.6 g/dl
WCC	15 x 10^9/l (neutrophils 40%, lymphocytes 38%, monocytes 12%, basophils 3%, eosinophils 1%, atypical lymphocytes 6%)
Platelets	15 x 10^9/l
Blood film	Normal apart from thrombocytopenia
Karyotype on blood	Unsuccessful
Karyotype on marrow cells	Showed the original abnormality t (3;11;13) with an isochromosome 17 in all 20 cells examined

The patient was treated with hydroxyurea, 1 g daily, and entered a stable chronic phase with a normal blood count. Eighteen months later she complained of frontal headaches and intermittent visual blurring. Examination was unremarkable and showed a normal-sized spleen and normal fundi. Results of her blood count and karyotype tests are shown in **122**.

Questions h, i
h What is the differential diagnosis?
i What further tests would you advise?

Grey case 25 (Part 1)

A 71-year-old man presented with painful dusky blue ischaemic toes; the tip of the left fifth toe had become black. Although the symptoms in his toes had been present for only four weeks, he had had intermittent claudication in both calves for three years. On mild exertion he became dyspnoeic, he smoked 25 cigarettes daily, and in the winter was prone to bronchitis. He drank 30 units of beer a week.

On examination he was 85 kg, apyrexial, and did not appear cyanosed. Clubbing and lymphadenopathy were not detected. Respiratory examination revealed a hyperinflated chest with a few coarse creps at the right lung base. His pulse was 78/min sinus rhythm and blood pressure 145/90 mm Hg. Abdominal examination was normal. Neither foot felt cold, neither posterior tibial nor dorsalis pedis pulses could be felt. Toes on both feet were cold and blue with minimal capillary flow. The left fifth toe was gangrenous. Results of initial investigations are shown (**123**).

123

Test	Result	Normal
Hb	17.0 g/dl	
Haematocrit	0.48	
WCC	9.8 x 10^9/l	
Platelets	548 x 10^9/l	
ESR	70 mm/hr	
Blood film	Normal apart from a few target cells	
U&Es	Normal	
Blood gases		
PO$_2$	9.5 kPa	12–15
pCO$_2$	4.3 kPa	4.4–6.1
H$^+$	37 nmol/l	36–44
Bicarbonate	28 mmol/l	24–30

Questions a–c
a Discuss these results.
b Suggest differential diagnoses.
c List further pertinent investigations.

Grey case 25 (Part 2)

Questions d, e
d In view of the results of further investigations (124), what is the probable haematological diagnosis?

e What management would you institute?

Test	Result	Normal	124
Red cell mass	0.034l/kg	0.028–0.035	
Plasma volume	0.041l/kg	0.040–0.050	
Bleeding time (template)	9 mins	Up to 8	
Platelet aggregation			
ADP	Normal		
Collagen	Normal		
Ristocetin	Normal		
Adrenaline	Absent		
Abdominal ultrasound	Liver normal texture and size; spleen 5 cm	8–14	
Urate	0.45 mmol/l	0.12–0.42	

Grey case 26 (Part 1)

A 65-year-old Greek lady presented with a three-month history of easy bruising. She also reported a left-sided stabbing chest pain on exertion, which was not relieved by sublingual GTN. Her medication was atenolol 50 mg daily and GTN as required. Past medical history included a hernia repair and cholecystectomy at the age of 31. The patient is married, her husband is a miner, and she is a retired cook. She has not smoked for the past 10 years, but drinks about 10–20 units of alcohol a week.

The only significant findings on examination were petechiae around both ankles and scattered, non-tender bruises, mainly on the shins and lower arms. The results of initial investigations are shown in 125.

Questions a, b
a What is the most likely diagnosis?

b What treatment is appropriate?

Test	Result	125
Hb	10.7 g/dl (MCV103 fl; MCH 32.0 pg)	
WCC	3.1 x 10⁹/l(48% neutrophils)	
Platelets	12 x 10⁹/l	
Peripheral blood film	Macrocytes and thrombocytopenia	
Sternal bone marrow aspirate	Hypercellular; occasional micromegakaryocytes and sideroblasts	
Coagulation screen	Normal	
U&Es	Normal	
Liver function tests	Normal	
Autoantibody screen	Negative	
B$_{12}$	400 ng/l (120–600)	
Serum folate	3.1 µg/l (1.6–6.0)	

Grey case 26 (Part 2)

Over the next two years, the patient required regular treatment with platelet concentrates and occasional blood cell transfusions. Infection was not a problem. It was noted that towards the end of this period, the patient was becoming more transfusion dependent. About two years after the first presentation, after direct questioning by the SHO, the patient admitted to a several week history of dark urine and vague abdominal pains. A typical FBC at that time revealed:

- Hb 8.2 g/dl;
- WCC 3.6 x 10^9/l;
- platelets 83 x 10^9/l.

Questions c, d
c What investigations are required now?
d What diagnoses would you consider?

Grey case 26 (Part 3)

126

Test	Result	Normal
U&Es	Normal	
Calcium	2.03 mmol/l	2.2–2.6
Albumin	23 g/l	35–50
Alk phosph	319 iu/l	30–115
AST	50 iu/l	5-45
Bilirubin	39 μmol/l	0–17
One stage PT	39.6 secs	14.2
Thrombin clotting time	16.2 secs	13.8
KCCT	41.4 secs	39.2
Radiograph of knee joints	Intra-articular calcification	

The patient was treated with folic acid and short courses of steroids, which did little to help the peripheral blood picture. She continued to have repeated episodes of intravascular haemolysis, requiring repeated blood transfusions.

Two years later, the patient suffered further abdominal pain, became jaundiced, and complained of joint pains in the shoulders and knees. Investigations that were considered to be relevant, were performed and the results are shown in **126**.

Questions e–g
e What is likely to have happened?
f What further tests are required?
g What course of action can be taken?

Grey case 27

A 5-year-old girl was seen in clinic suffering from palpitations. Examination and routine investigations were normal. Three months later she presented with dyspnoea and sweats. Examination revealed signs of a pericardial effusion and hepatosplenomegaly. Results of investigations are shown in **127**.

Questions a, b
a Discuss the differential diagnosis.
b Discuss the further investigation of this child.

Test	Result	127
FBC	Normal	
Pericardio-centesis	Straw-coloured fluid, containing lymphoid cells	
Immuno-phenotype of these cells		
CD2	91%	
CD3	3%	
CD7	1%	
CD10	31%	
CD19	82%	
CD45	90%	
Tdt	17%	
Cyt IgM	2%	
Cytogenetics of the cells	42, XX, -2, -5, -6, -9, -11, -13, -17, -18, t(6;18), t(9;19), t(11;13) in 15/30 cells examined	
Bone marrow aspirate	Normal morphology, but cytogenetics revealed the cytogenetic abnormality	
Repeat bone marrow 2 weeks later	20% abnormal cells (**128**)	

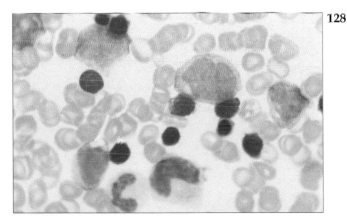

128

Grey case 28

129

Test	Result	Normal
Hb	5.5 g/l (fragmented erythrocytes present)	
Reticulocytes	21%	
WCC	15.5x10⁹/l (neutrophilia)	
Platelets	40 x 10⁹/l	
APTT	39 secs	28–38
PT	16 secs	13–16
Fibrinogen	1.6 g/l	1.5–4.0
U&Es	Normal	

An 18-year-old girl was admitted as an emergency feeling faint and with lower abdominal pain. Her last menstrual period was 14 weeks previously. She had not attended any antenatal clinic.

On examination she looked unwell and pale; her temperature was 38.2°C. Her pulse was 92/min sinus rhythm with a BP of 105/60 mm Hg. Abdominal examination revealed hypogastric tenderness and a mass arising from the pelvis. An ultrasound scan confirmed an enlarged uterus and revealed that it contained a dead fetus.

The results of initial investigations are shown in **129**.

Questions a, b, c

a What are the most likely diagnoses?

b What immediate management would be appropriate?

c What will you tell the patient about the possibility of her having a recurrence during her next pregnancy?

Grey cases: answers

Grey case 1 (Part 1 a–c)

a The diagnosis is:
- acute myeloblastic leukaemia. The confusional state may be due to intracerebral bleeding (which could be related to a coagulation disturbance) or hyperleucocytosis (which is more common in M4 and M5 disease).

b Essential further investigations are:
- coagulation screen, to include prothrombin time, partial thromboplastin time, plasma fibrinogen, and a measure of fibrinogen degradation products;
- further studies on the blast cells including immunophenotype and cytogenetics.

c Treatment needed is as follows.
- Reduce the peripheral blood blast cell count immediately using a cell separator.
- Transfuse platelets, but not blood (patients with hyperleucocytosis are usually protected from hyperviscosity syndrome by anaemia; blood transfusion may result in lethargy, visual disturbances and coma).
- Further treatment with fresh frozen plasma and possibly heparin if the coagulation screen indicates disseminated intravascular coagulation.
- Consider starting specific chemotherapy to treat the acute leukaemia.

Grey case 1 (Part 2 d–f)

d In view of the long period of neutropenia, systemic fungal infection with lung involvement is the most likely diagnosis. Other possibilities include *Pneumocystis* pneumonia and cytomegalovirus (CMV). Other viral pneumonias are possible, but less likely.

e Additional investigations.
- Further cultures of blood and sputum (if available) for bacteria and fungi.
- Tests of pulmonary function including blood gases.
- Bronchoscopy and bronchial lavage for fungal spores, *Pneumocystis*, and CMV. (Note there is a low rate of positive cultures for CMV.)
- Consider transbronchial lung biopsy with platelet transfusion cover. This is often the only way to resolve differential diagnostic difficultion of this type.

f Further treatment indicated is as follows.
- Start intravenous amphotericin to a maximum dose of 1 mg/kg/day (care needed with renal function) for presumed fungal infection.
- Add co-trimoxazole (high-dose) 120 mg/kg/day in divided doses to treat possible *Pneumocystis carinii*.
- Change broad-spectrum antibiotics.
- Consider artificial ventilation.

Grey case 2 (Part 1 a)

a The antithrombin III level is markedly reduced. This suggests congenital antithrombin III deficiency. However, heparin therapy itself can lower the level and may be the explanation. The protein C level is within the normal range, which extends down to levels that might be considered as pathological for other coagulation inhibitors.

The protein C level increases with age, but levels in the region of 68% are within the normal age-specific range for a 25-year-old female. The free protein S level is reduced, probably due to the oral contraceptive. This and pregnancy are associated with lower concentrations.

Grey case 2 (Part 2 b, c)

b The antithrombin III level is still reduced in the absence of heparin providing more evidence for congenital antithrombin III deficiency. The protein C and S levels are reduced. This is because both are vitamin K-dependent proteins and their concentrations fall in patients on warfarin.

c Warfarin should be continued for a total of six months. A further citrated blood sample should be obtained two months after stopping warfarin.

Grey case 2 (Part 3 d, e)

d The antithrombin III activity level remains low, but the antigen concentrate is normal. This patient therefore has type II antithrombin III deficiency. The protein C and S are now both normal.

e It is necessary to consider whether or not this patient should be on long-term warfarin therapy. As she has only had a single deep vein thrombosis (DVT) that might have been precipitated by the oral contraceptive it would be reasonable to withhold warfarin. If, however, she develops a further DVT without provocation, there would be a stronger argument for starting long-term warfarin. The patient will need to be advised that there is an increased risk of developing a DVT if she becomes pregnant. During subsequent pregnancies she should receive subcutaneous heparin. There are no firm guidelines about the use of antithrombin concentrates in pregnancy. Although some would recommend starting regular infusions at 32 weeks' gestation, others would give the concentrate just over the delivery period and continue it for several days after delivery until the patient is fully warfarinised. Warfarin should then be continued for six months. As antithrombin III deficiency is an autosomal dominant disorder, it is important to screen the patient's parents and siblings for the deficiency.

Grey case 3 (Part 1 a–c)

a A reasonable diagnosis would be gastroenteritis.

b Initial investigations would include a FBC, urea and electrolytes, blood cultures, stool culture, and microscopy. The results are shown in **130**.

c Management would consist of rehydration with intravenous fluids, antiemetics, and antidiarrhoeal agents.

Test	Result	130
Hb	15.2 g/dl	
WCC	20.7 x 10⁹/l with a neutrophilia	
Platelets	130 x 10⁹/l	
Sodium	136 mmol/l	
Potassium	3.5 mmol/l	
Urea	5.4 mmol/l	
Creatinine	95 µmol/l	
Stool and blood cultures to date	Negative	

Grey case 3 (Part 2 d, e)

d The differential diagnosis must now include:
- septicaemia with disseminated intravascular coagulation (DIC);
- idiopathic thrombocytopenic purpura;
- haemolytic uraemic syndrome (HUS) /thrombotic thrombocytopenic purpura (TTP);
- inflammatory bowel disease;
- persistent gastroenteritis.

e Further useful investigations include examination of the blood film, repeat urea and electrolytes, DIC screen, and bone marrow examination.

Grey case 3 (Part 3 f–h)

f The most likely diagnosis is HUS precipitated by gastroenteritis. The most common pathogen in the UK that causes this condition is *E. coli* 0157.

g *E. coli* 0157 can be looked for in the stool, but it is possible using an ELISA technique to detect serum antibodies to it. In this patient, this test was positive with a result of 1.34 units (a negative result being less than 0.5 units).

h The treatment of this condition is daily plasmapheresis with a 3-litre exchange and replacement with FFP.

Renal function and blood pressure must be closely monitored. This patient did, in fact, become hypertensive, and this was successfully controlled with a combination of atenolol and nifedipine. Within a few days, renal function showed signs of improvement and had returned to normal. The patient's condition has otherwise completely improved, though she continues antihypertensive medication for the time being.

Grey case 4 (Part 1 a, b)

a The blood film shows hypochromic microcytic red cells with marked anisocytosis and poikilocytosis. There are many target cells and there is red cell polychromasia. The diagnosis is likely to be β-thalassaemia major.

b Hb electrophoresis is required (HbA2 not detected, HbF 92% confirming the diagnosis of β-thalassaemia major).

Grey case 4 (Part 2 c, d)

c The well-maintained physical state and reasonably good Hb indicates that this boy's β-thalassaemia major is running a 'benign' course; this is called β-thalassaemia intermedia. Frontal bossing and maxillary expansion suggests medullary expansion due to ineffective erythropoiesis. Splenomegaly suggests increasing extramedullary haematopoiesis.

d The clinical phenotype of β-thalassaemia intermedia falls between that of the transfusion-dependent thalassaemia major and the asymptomatic thalassaemia minor (trait) and individuals usually maintain a Hb of 7 g/dl or greater. In homozygous β-thalassaemia this may be due to co-inheritance of α-thalassaemia, enhanced production of HbF, or a β-globin mutation causing a mild decrease in β–globin expression.

Grey case 4 (Part 3 e–g)

e Despite increasing medullary expansion (ribs) and extramedullary haematopoiesis (liver and spleen) the patient is failing to maintain his Hb and he requires blood transfusion.
f Further investigations required include:
• urea and electrolytes (normal);
• ALT 10 iu/l (5–45 iu/l);
• ALP 470 iu/l (30–115 iu/l);
• albumin 35 g/l (35–50 g/l);
• bilirubin 16 μmol/l (1–17 μmol/l);
• serum ferritin 285 μg/l (15–300μg/l);
• full red cell genotyping.

g Management now is as follows.
• The patient needs to embark on a hypertransfusion regimen aiming for a mean Hb of 12 g/dl. This requires transfusion to maintain Hb above 10 g/dl to a maximum of 15 g/dl. Blood should be leucocyte-depleted, either by in-line filtration or by using washed red cells resuspended in saline. Leucocyte depletion decreases the development of HLA-associated antibodies, which are a major cause of non-haemolytic transfusion reactions in multiply transfused individuals.

- The serum ferritin must be monitored with the intention of commencing desferrioxamine iron chelation therapy when it reaches 500–1000 µg/l. The usual method of chelation is by overnight subcutaneous infusion of desferrioxamine via a pump mechanism and in addition intravenous desferrioxamine may be given concurrently with blood transfusion. Patients (particularly children) find that a long indwelling intravenous catheter (e.g. Port-A-Cath) is advantageous. Vitamin C (ascorbic acid) increases the efficacy of iron chelation by desferrioxamine.
- Folic acid supplementation is required because folate demands are high.
- Monitoring for side-effects of desferrioxamine chelation, including annual ophthalmological and audiological assessment. Desferrioxamine will chelate some trace metals and zinc deficiency may occur.
- In the long term, the effects of iron overload will need to be monitored.

Grey case 5 (Part 1 a–c)

a The differential diagnosis is:
- graft versus host disease (liver and gut), but the absence of a skin rash is unusual and the timing (day 8 post BMT) is early, especially after a T cell-depleted transplant;
- bacterial septicaemia;
- fungal septicaemia (unlikely at this stage);

b FBC, film, bone marrow aspirate, liver function tests, renal function tests, blood cultures. The results are shown in 131.

c Broad-spectrum intravenous antibiotics for bacterial infection. Vancomycin or teicoplanin will be required to treat the staphylococcal infection. Consider high-dose steroids (methylprednisolone intravenously) for graft versus host disease. Maintain good hydration.

131

Test	Result
Hb	10.2 g/dl
WCC	0.1 x 10^9/l
Platelets	10 x 10^9/l
Film	Occasional lymphocytes seen
Bone marrow aspirate	Occasional early normoblasts and a rare megakaryocyte, but no evidence of myelopoiesis
Serum bilirubin	80 µmol/l (normal 1–17)
Alkaline phosphatase	306 iu/l (normal 30–115)
Liver enzymes	Normal
Renal function	Normal
Blood cultures	Grew *Staphylococcus epidermidis* in three separate samples

Grey case 5 (Part 2 d–f)

d Additional diagnoses to consider are:
- veno-occlusive disease of the liver;
- untreated infection;
- disseminated intravascular coagulation (DIC);
- thrombotic thrombocytopenic purpura (TTP).

e Blood urea (9.6 mmol/l), serum creatinine (170 µmol/l), DIC screen (normal), stool cultures (negative).

f Change antibiotics. Use antibiotics which are not nephrotoxic in view of the minor abnormalities in renal function. Consider removing the Hickman line, which is almost certainly colonised with *Staph. epidermidis*.

Grey case 5 (Part 3 g–i)

g The patient has hepatic veno-occlusive disease of the liver.

h Definitive diagnosis is very difficult and would be confirmed only by a liver biopsy, which in this case would not be recommended in view of the persistently low platelet count.

i Predisposing factors include:
- conditioning regimens which contain high dose busulphan;
- previous liver disease;
- the use of hepatotoxic drugs;
- high tumour burden (not relevant here).

Grey case 6 (a, b)

a The differential diagnosis is as follows.
- Idiopathic myelofibrosis. This is extremely rare in childhood, most cases being associated with acute leukaemia, marrow involvement with solid tumour, viral infection, or myelodysplasia. In this context, the diagnosis of acute megakaryoblastic leukaemia (AML M7) should be considered, but the platelet marker CD42 was negative, and further study with platelet-specific markers (platelet peroxidase, anti-von Willebrand factor) would be needed to substantiate this diagnosis. Myelofibrosis is sometimes associated with acute lymphoblastic leukaemia, but the cell markers do not indicate this diagnosis.

• An alternative diagnosis would be myelofibrotic myelodysplasia. The marrow cytogenetics indicate that there are four chromosome 21s. Children with Down's syndrome typically have trisomy 21, and so there is an extra chromosome 21 present in the abnormal clone. An extra chromosome 21 is a recognised finding in AML M7, but has also been described in ALL.

From the information provided, a differential diagnosis of myelofibrosis associated with myelodysplasia (RAEB) or AML is likely, but the data are insufficient for a more precise conclusion.

b Down's syndrome may be associated with a leukaemoid reaction in the newborn period, an increased incidence of acute lymphoid and myeloid leukaemia, myelodysplasia, and neonatal polycythaemia.

Grey case 7 (Part 1 a, b)

a The anaemia is probably secondary to bleeding into the thigh. The APTT is prolonged and is only partially corrected by normal plasma. It is likely, therefore, that he has a circulatory inhibitor of his coagulation system. In the presence of an haemorrhagic state the most likely would be an antifactor VIII antibody.

b A factor VIII and vWF assay and if low an assessment of the concentration of the inhibitor.

Grey case 7 (Part 2 c, d)

c The factor VIII level is reduced and an apparent low level inhibitor is present. In acquired haemophilia it is usual for the factor VIII level to be reduced to less than 0.01 iu/ml and for the patient to present with spontaneous bruising and haematomas. However, some spontaneously arising anti-factor VIII antibodies do not completely inactivate circulating factor VIII activity.

d The patient should be treated with factor VIII concentrate. Thereafter serial blood samples should be collected to assess the recovery of factor VIII *in vivo* and its half-life within the circulation.

Grey case 7 (Part 3 e, f)

e The post-infusion factor VIII level is less than anticipated in the absence of an inhibitor. In a man such as this, without an inhibitor, 43 U/kg should give a post-infusion level of approximately 1.00 iu/ml. The recovery is therefore only approximately 20% of that anticipated. Furthermore, the half-life of the infused factor VIII is less than 2 hours; this is much shorter than the normal of about 12 hours. This data therefore supports the presence of an anti-factor VIII inhibitor.

f Regular three times daily factor VIII infusions should be given. It is likely that after several infusions the recovery and half-life of the transfused factor VIII will increase as the inhibitor is neutralised. Thereafter it will therefore be possible to use smaller doses.

Factor VIII recoveries should be measured regularly to ensure that adequate factor levels are being maintained and that the inhibitor is not undergoing an anamnestic response. Although this is characteristic of anti-factor VIII inhibitors arising in individuals with congenital haemophilia, it is uncommon in those with acquired haemophilia. If the level of inhibitor rises, its reactivity against porcine factor VIII should be assessed as it may have only a low level of cross-reactivity. The infusions of factor VIII should be continued until the haematoma has resolved. In older patients the inhibitors are rather more persistent and cyclophosphamide 100 mg/day should be given a therapeutic trial.

Grey case 8 (Part 1 a, b)

a The differential diagnosis is obviously diabetes mellitus, which may account for the peripheral neuropathy, and in addition, there is evidence of chronic liver disease, providing a differential diagnosis of:
- cirrhosis of either alcoholic or hepatic aetiology;
- porphyria cutanea tarda;
- haemochromatosis.

In addition, he could have carcinoma of the bowel or lung, with peripheral neuropathy as a non-metastatic manifestation of malignant disease.

b Investigations required are:
- FBC;
- ultrasound of abdomen;
- urea and electrolytes;
- ferritin;
- liver function tests;
- chest radiograph;
- urinary porphyrins;
- blood glucose capillary series;
- liver biopsy.

Grey case 8 (Part 2 c)

c Other investigations that would be most useful are:
- serum iron (28 μmol/l (10–35 μmol/l);
- TIBC 28.5 μmol/l (35–70 μmol/l).

Transferrin saturation is therefore almost 100%.

Grey case 8 (Part 3 d, e)

d The diagnosis is haemochromatosis.
e The treatment is regular venesection. Screening of other family members by measurement of serum iron and TIBC should be considered.The patient was regularly venesected one unit/week. It took two years for the transferrin saturation to fall to less than 50%. This is strongly suggestive of haemochromatosis. Transferrin saturation and ferritin may be high initially in alcoholic haemosiderosis. Regular venesection produces a sharp fall in these parameters to normal values, since the amount of iron deposited is generally much less than in haemochromatosis. His diabetes mellitus was subsequently controlled on insulin, but he did develop proliferative retinopathy, which required laser treatment.

Grey case 8 (Part 4 f–h)

f He has developed polycythaemia.
g Blood volume estimations need to be carried out, which showed a true erythrocytosis with a normal plasma volume.

h The likely aetiological factors in this man are alcohol and chronic liver disease, and hypoxia secondary to chronic obstructive airways disease.

Grey case 8 (Part 5 i, j)

i The differential diagnosis is cirrhosis, alcoholic hepatitis, or hepatoma.
j Other tests would include:
- abdominal ultrasound, which showed multiple hypoechoic foci consistent with malignancy;

- INR (1.1);
- alpha feta protein, which was elevated at 325 U/l;
- ultrasound-guided liver biopsy, which demonstrated hepatocellular carcinoma and micronodular cirrhosis.

Grey case 9 (Part 1 a, b)

a The differential diagnosis must include acute myeloid leukaemia (rash and organomegaly) and acute lymphoblastic leukaemia.

b Initial investigations would include FBC, biochemistry, a bone marrow aspirate, and cytogenetics.

Grey case 9 (Part 2 c, d)

c The diagnosis is juvenile-chronic myeloid leukaemia (J-CML).

d This condition usually responds well to treatment with hydroxyurea, but unfortunately there was no response to this in either WCC or organomegaly. His treatment was therefore changed to 6 mercaptopurine.

Grey case 9 (Part 3 e, f)

e The blood film shows tear drop poikilocytes, nucleated red cells, and left shifted granulocytes.

f Further investigations required are:
● a differential WCC;
● bone marrow aspirate;
● bone marrow trephine biopsy;
● cytogenetic studies.

Grey case 9 (Part 4 g–i)

g The bone marrow aspirate shows increased numbers of left shifted megakaryocytes; normal myelopoiesis (3% eosinophils and occasional basophils, no blasts); normoblastic erythropoiesis with tear drop poikilocytes (J-CML in remission ?myelofibrosis). The bone marrow trephine shows a hypercellular marrow, myeloid hyperplasia with increased megakaryocytes, no blast transformation, and marked increase in reticulin deposition (i.e. J-CML transformed to myelofibrosis).

h This child has developed myelofibrosis, almost certainly as a consequence of his initial J-CML. His liver and spleen will be important sites of extramedullary haematopoiesis. In addition he has hypersplenic features (i.e. thrombocytopenia and enlarging spleen size after blood transfusion associated with poor Hb increment).

i A liver biopsy was taken (**132**), which demonstrated extramedullary haematopoiesis and some fibrosis. Aims in management are:

- reversal of myelofibrosis by further 6-mercaptopurine treatment to improve marrow haematopoiesis;
- reduction of splenic bulk by 6-MP or more aggressive chemotherapy or local radiotherapy;
- splenectomy.

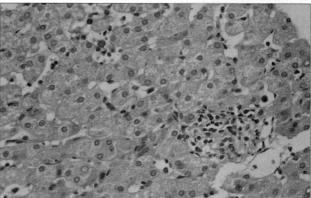

132

The concern is that the spleen is an important site of extramedullary haematopoiesis and if removed may result in relentless hepatomegaly. An attempt should be made to improve the status of the marrow by intensive chemotherapy with or without bone marrow transplantation to offer some hope of long-term survival.

Grey case 10 (Part 1 a–e)

a Aplastic anaemia.

b Bone marrow aspirate and trephine. The aspirate produced a 'dry tap' with very few identifiable cells. The trephine showed an empty marrow with occasional plasma cells and normal lymphocytes, but no identifiable erythroid or myeloid precursors and no megakaryocytes.

c Chloramphenicol eye drops.

d The severe irreversible type of chloramphenicol aplasia can occur long after finishing treatment. The mechanism is unclear, but is generally believed to be dose-dependent. There is no existing test for chloramphenicol-induced aplasia. The evidence in the literature is purely epidemiological.

e Chloramphenicol aplasia is generally irreversible and the usual treatments (e.g. methylprednisolone, anti-lymphocyte (or thymocyte) globulin, cyclosporin) are ineffective. The preferred treatment in this young patient is early bone marrow transplantation. Blood transfusions (red cells and platelets) should be leucocyte-depleted. Blood transfusion from family members greatly increases the risk of rejection and should be avoided.

Grey case 10 (Part 2 f–i)

f Paroxysmal nocturnal haemoglobinuria (PNH). The relationship between aplasia and PNH is complex, but PNH complicates aplasia in the early or late stages in up to 25% of survivors. The likely cause is the development by somatic mutation, of a clone of stem cells with a biological advantage over remaining stem cells and producing the dyohaematopoietic cells of PNH. The change seems particularly likely in patients whose marrow injury has a toxic aetiology (e.g. chloramphenicol).

g PNH cells are unusually susceptible to lysis by complement and a positive Ham's acidified serum lysis test is probably the best method, but this phenomenon can be demonstrated by sucrose, thrombin, insulin, cobra-venom and cold-antibody lysis tests. Haemoglobin and haemosiderin can be demonstrated in the patient's urine.

h It is probably adequate to replace lysed red cells by transfusion of filtered washed red cells. Androgens and prednisolone have been tried, but often without effect. Bone marrow transplantation has been successful in severe cases.

i Matched unrelated donor bone marrow transplantation.

Grey case 10 (Part 3 j–l)

j Chronic graft versus host disease (GVHD) of the lung. Chronic GVHD occurs in about 40% of patients following a bone marrow transplant and is commoner in patients who have had significant acute GVHD. Cytomegalovirus infection has its peak incidence at about this time and can be confused with chronic GVHD. In this case, the diagnosis was confirmed by lung biopsy.

k General supportive care with oxygen administration. Intravenous high-dose methylprednisolone with reducing dosage as the patient responds.

l Scleroderma, which is an occasional manifestation of chronic skin GVHD. Treatment is difficult, but some response has been seen to cyclosporin, oral prednisolone, azathioprine, or thalidomide.

Grey case 11

a The investigations indicate a leucoery-throblastic anaemia, with associated thrombocytopenia. The bone marrow appearances are consistent with either a myeloproliferative disorder or peripheral destruction of cells with compensatory marrow hyperplasia. The presence of minor dysplastic features does not distinguish between a primary or reactive marrow disorder. Causes of gross splenomegaly in childhood include leukaemia, myeloproliferative disease, portal hypertension, and storage disorders. Lesser degrees of splenomegaly are associated with congenital and acquired infection, haemolysis, autoimmune disorders, immune deficiency, and vascular malformations. There was no evidence of liver disease in this child, but specific investigations to exclude these possibilities are indicated. Marrow cytogenetics were normal, but this does not exclude a myeloproliferative disorder.

b HbF should be measured to exclude juvenile CGL, although the WCC was not elevated. The immunoglobulins were abnormal, with low IgG and mildly elevated IgM. Although hepatosplenomegaly may be a feature of immune deficiency, the low IgG may be a secondary change.

Grey case 12 (Part 1 a, b)

a The differential diagnosis is:
• idiopathic thrombocytopenic purpura;
• mild pre-eclampsia;
• HELLP syndrome;
• congenital thrombocytopenia;
• marrow infiltration.

b Further investigations should include bone marrow aspirate, coagulation screen, urinary protein/24 hours, serum urate, urea and electrolytes, liver function tests, Coomb's test, viral titres, autoantibodies.

Grey case 12 (Part 2 c, d)

c The lack of evidence for pre-eclampsia and the normal coagulation screen make this diagnosis unlikely as the cause of thrombocytopenia. Although the ALT is marginally raised the bilirubin is normal as are the reticulocytes making a diagnosis of HELLP unlikely. The absence of infiltrate in the marrow aspirate makes it unlikely the patient had thrombocytopenia secondary to malignancy in the marrow. The patient is therefore likely to have ITP or a congenital thrombocytopenia. This latter diagnosis is unlikely because it is rare and the platelet morphology was normal. The most likely diagnosis, despite the absence of autoantibodies or evidence of viral infection is ITP.

d No therapy is needed whilst her platelet count remains above 50 x 10^9/l. She should have weekly platelet counts and if the platelets fall below this level the choice is between prednisolone and intravenous immunoglobulin. Both are likely to give a reasonable increment to her platelets. As she is nearing the end of her pregnancy, after which her platelet count may return spontaneously to normal, it would be reasonable to avoid steroids and give intravenous immunoglobulin (1–2 g/kg). Alternatively she should be started on prednisolone 40mg/day; careful monitoring of her blood pressure will be required in view of its current level.Provided her platelet count is above $50 \times 10^9/1$ it is probably

reasonable to allow pregnancy to proceed to term and a spontaneous vaginal delivery. There is a chance the fetus will be thrombocytopenic due to the presumed anti-platelet antibody crossing the placenta. If a difficult labour is anticipated, therefore, a Caesarean section might be more appropriate to reduce potential trauma to the fetus. Mild to moderately thrombocytopenic mothers usually have few bleeding problems following delivery but haemorrhage from the episiotomy site is not uncommon. The platelet count of the baby should be measured immediately after birth.

Grey case 13 (Part 1 a, b)

a The differential diagnosis must include acute lymphoblastic leukaemia, acute myeloid leukaemia, Fanconi's anaemia and severe aplastic anaemia.
b Investigations required are:
• biochemistry;

• bone marrow aspiration;
• bone marrow trephine;
• blood chromosomes;
• HbF;
• viral studies;
• skeletal survey.

Grey case 13 (Part 2 c, d)

c The diagnosis is idiopathic severe aplastic anaemia. The microcephaly, low birth weight, and neonatal failure to thrive are suggestive of a constitutional predisposition, but specific investigations of chromosomal fragility were normal, ruling out Fanconi's anaemia. There is no apparent viral aetiology.
d Management in the first instance is supportive with red cell and platelet transfusions usually having inserted a permanent intravenous line. These

products should be given via leucocyte depleting filters to minimize HLA antigen exposure. The curative procedure for this boy would be early allogeneic bone marrow transplantation. He is however an only child, therefore excluding sibling transplant; other treatment alternatives are:
• immunosuppression with antithymocyte globulin (horse or rabbit) ± steroids ± cyclosporin A± androgens (e.g. oxymetholone).

Grey case 13 (Part 3 e–g)

e Disseminated fungal infection is the most likely cause of which, with a history of pleuritic chest pain, *Aspergillus* is the most likely. Swabs from this lesion produced a profuse growth of *Aspergillus flavus*.

f He was treated with intravenous amphotericin B, which was changed to a liposomal formulation to escalate the dose to 5 mg/kg/day.

g Deep-seated fungal infection in a patient with no expectation of spontaneous recovery of neutrophil numbers requires long-term antifungal therapy. Further immunosuppressive therapy for severe aplastic anaemia is likely to be complicated by a recrudescence of fungal infection. He would be a very high-risk patient in view of his infection history and numbers of blood products already received for an unrelated donor bone marrow transplantation. The best option is probably to attempt a second course of ATG (rabbit) with anti-*Aspergillus* therapy (e.g. itraconazole or liposomal amphotericin B).

Grey case 14

a There is an extensive yellow-brown macular rash, typical of Langerhan cell histiocytosis (histiocytosis X). A clinical presentation with otorrhoea, rash, lymphadenopathy, and hepatosplenomegaly is typical of the multi-organ form of the disease, which affects very young children. The pancytopenia suggests bone marrow involvement.

b Further investigations include the following.

• A full assessment of the extent of the disease with skeletal survey, bone marrow aspirate and trephine, chest radiography, and liver function tests.

• Diagnostic confirmation by skin biopsy with a demonstration of a histiocytic or lymphohistiocytic infiltrate. It is crucial to demonstrate the characteristics of Langerhan's cells in the histiocytes. These include Birbeck granules on electron microscopy, and positivity for S100 protein, CD1, and staining with alpha-mannosidase and peanut agglutinin.

c Treatment for multisystem disease includes immunosuppression, most commonly with corticosteroids, and vinblastine or etoposide. There are cases with at least partial response to cyclosporin.

d The prognosis for infants with multisystem disease is poor, with 60% mortality due to organ failure and intercurrent infection.

Grey case 15 (Part 1 a–c)

a The presence of the antibodies can be explained by the history of previous transfusion and previous pregnancies.

b Further testing is indicated. Both mother and father should be genotyped and the anti-D antibody should be quantified. It is also possible in specialist centres to determine blood group at 12 weeks' gestation by chorionic villous biopsy, or from 18 weeks onwards by fetal blood sampling. The haemolytic potential of the anti-D can be assessed by macrophage phagocytosis assay or an antibody-dependent cell-mediated cytotoxic assay, which appears to correlate more closely with clinical outcome than the anti-D level *per se*. In this case, the genotype of the mother was rrkk and the genotype of the father was R2rkk.

c The mother should be reviewed at monthly intervals.

Grey case 15 (Part 2 d)

d Amniocentesis is indicated at 24 weeks' gestation (i.e., when the anti-D is 4 IU/ml). It is worth noting that this baby may have an R2 phenotype, which is more susceptible to haemolytic disease than R1 phenotype.

Grey case 15 (Part 3 e, f)

e Induction of labour should be considered at 35 weeks.

f Amniocentesis can also determine the lecithin/sphingomyelin ratio, which should be greater than 2 for safe induction.

Grey case 15 (Part 4 g–i)

g The Hb and bilirubin indicate that the baby should receive an exchange transfusion.

h The anti-Kell is unlikely to be contributory to the haemolytic disease of the newborn, since both mother and father are Kell-negative. Unless there is a problem with paternity, the baby should also be Kell-negative. The Kell phenotype of the baby can be easily checked. The presence of the anti-Kell on the baby's red cells is due to IgG placental transfer.

i There is no point in administering anti-D immunoglobulin to the mother.

Grey case 16 (Part 1 a, b)

a The differential diagnosis is:
- myelofibrosis. (Features in support are the patient's age, leucoerythroblastic anaemia and red cell and platelet morphology. Massive splenomegaly does not usually occur in the early stages of myelofibrosis and peripheral blood WBC is only modestly raised.)
- chronic myeloid leukaemia. (Patient's age, the absence of basophils and the pronounced red cell changes are not typical.)

b Further investigations indicated are:
- bone marrow trephine;
- karyotype;
- BCR gene rearrangement;
- serum folic acid;
- serum vitamin B_{12}.

Grey case 16 (Part 2 c)

c Treatment with alpha-interferon, which often has a selective effect on the platelet count may be used. Alternatives are other cytotoxic drugs such as busulphan or mitobronitol (also often platelet suppressive), but these drugs are less likely to be of use in this situation. Splenectomy is contraindicated especially in view of the high platelet count. If platelet adhesiveness is reduced using agents such as aspirin the risk of thrombosis is less.

Grey case 16 (Part 3 d)

d The differential diagnosis is:
- *Candida* oesophagitis. Barium swallow and oesophagoscopy were normal, excluding this diagnosis.
- Splenic infarction. Specific investigations to confirm this diagnosis are lacking, but the clinical situation makes the diagnosis unlikely (spleen size reducing on treatment, absence of splenic pain or splenic rub).
- Myocardial infarction (MI). Electrocardiogram showed evidence of a recent myocardial infarction. (Note that serum transaminases often rise in the early weeks of alpha INF treatment and cannot be used as a guide to diagnosis of MI). MI occurs as a rare complication of alpha-INF treatment, especially in elderly individuals.

121

Grey case 17 (Part 1 a, b)

a The blood film confirms the anaemia and shows spherocytes and polychromasia. In addition there is active erythrophagocytosis.

b Further investigations required are:
- biochemistry;
- coagulation tests;
- a direct antiglobulin test;
- a reticulocyte count;
- blood cultures;
- virology titres;
- *Mycoplasma* titre;
- immunoglobulins.

Grey case 17 (Part 2 c, d)

c The patient has a cold autoimmune haemolytic anaemia with evidence of brisk intravascular haemolysis, demonstrated by clinical signs of haemolysis and a positive DAT. Plasma hand spectroscopy showed the presence of methaemalbumin. The Donath–Landsteiner test was positive and is diagnostic of paroxysmal cold haemoglobinuria. There was insufficient serum to determine anti-P specificity of the antibody. This antibody is a polyclonal IgG antibody with biphasic characteristics. It binds with red cells at below 20°C in the peripheral circulation causing lysis by complement fixation when red cells return to the warmer central circulation. The liver is an important site for destruction of complement-coated red cells because it has a larger concentration of complement receptor-bearing macrophages compared with the spleen.

d Treatment consisted of keeping the patient as warm as possible and transfusing with the most ABO and Rhesus-compatible red cells. Unfortunately the haemolytic process failed to settle and the Hb could not be maintained above 6.8 g/dl with reticulocytes in the order of 3–4%. He was started on oral prednisolone and folic acid with a quick and good response. Reticulocytes rose to 23% and he settled and no further transfusion was necessary. The steroids were gradually reduced when Hb reached 12.4 g/dl and reticulocytes were 1.5%.

Grey case 18 (Part 1 a, b)

a Repeat antibody Rhesus grouping and antibody screening of the mother confirmed that the mother was O Rh-positive with a negative antibody screen. ABO and Rhesus grouping of the baby revealed B Rh-positive. Direct Coomb's test on cord cells was 1+, Hb 10.7 g/dl, WCC 12.7 x 10^9/l, and platelets 19 x 10^9/l. Bilirubin was 80 µmol/l. Examination of the blood film revealed the presence of spherocytes. These results suggest ABO haemolytic disease of the newborn. It is possible that phototherapy to the baby may be required, but the necessity for exchange transfusion is rare.

b The mother is Rh-positive and therefore prophylactic anti-D is not required.

Grey case 18 (Part 2 c)

c Possible diagnoses are:
- alloimmune thrombocytopenia;
- SLE;
- anti-PLA[1] antibody;
- congenital thrombocytopenia.

Grey case 18 (Part 3 d–f)

d The most likely diagnosis is an anti-PLA[1] antibody with placental transfer from the mother.

e The anti-PLA[1] antibody may be demonstrated in the maternal serum by immunofluorescence or ELISA technique. Platelet typing of the mother should demonstrate her to be PLA[1]-negative, while both the father and the baby should be PLA[1]-positive. About 5% of such cases are accounted for by platelet specific antigens other than the PLA[1] system.

f The treatment for the baby is with PLA[1]-negative platelets or intravenous immunoglobulin.

Grey case 19

(a) The history suggests atypical infection, and investigation should include full blood count, blood cultures, virology—particularly for Epstein–Barr virus and cytomegalovirus, serology for toxoplasma and brucella. In view of her history of travel, Leishmania serology is indicated. Tuberculosis should also be considered within the differential diagnosis.

(b) The bone marrow aspirate shows Leishman–Donovan bodies. The diagnosis is therefore visceral Leishmaniasis (kala-azar). This disease is endemic throughout the Mediterranean, with transmission by infected sandfly bite. There is a variable incubation period, from several months to many years, with gradual onset of debility, fever, hepatosplenomegaly, and pancytopenia. Untreated, death usually ensues from the complications of pancytopenia. The diagnosis is best made on tissue samples, including bone marrow, liver or lymph node biopsy, or splenic needle aspirate. Serology may also be used to sustantiate the diagnosis. Treatment has relied on administration of pentavalent antimonial compounds, but resistance has been an increasing problem. Amphotericin B is effective in resistant cases, and liposomal Amphotericin has shown great promise in clinical trials. Pentamidine has been used as a second-line treatment, but other agents (Rifampicin, Co-trimoxazole, Allopurinol) are not recommended. Long-term follow-up is required due to the risk of relapse. This girl was treated with a 6-day course of liposomal Amphotericin, with good effect.

Grey case 20 (Part 1 a, b)

a She could have intra abdominal infection, possibly early peritonitis. The
cause of the marked thrombocytopenia is not immediately apparent.
The coagulation screen is in keeping
with developing DIC secondary to
possible septicaemia. She may have
developed a DVT. She might have
heparin-induced thrombocytopenia.

b Additional investigations required
are a venogram, plain abdominal
radio-graphs, chest radiograph, and
blood cultures.

Grey case 20 (Part 2 c, d)

c Mesenteric artery thrombosis is characteristic of heparin induced thrombocytopenia; the DVT may well also
have been precipitated by heparin.
No further unfractionated heparin
should be given. A caval filter should
be inserted to prevent embolisation.
An alternative anticoagulant is indicated. This could either be one of the
low molecular weight heparins, ancrod, or warfarin therapy.

d Heparin-induced thrombocytopenia
usually becomes apparent at 7–10
days following initiation of therapy. It
is therefore important to perform regular platelet counts on any patient receiving heparin for more than five
days. Thrombosis is a characteristic
feature and it is often arterial. It is essential to stop the heparin immediately and institute another form of
anticoagulation (e.g. low molecular
weight heparin, ancrod, tPA, streptok-
inase, or warfarin depending on the
clinical indication).

Grey case 21 (Part 1 a, b)

a Sarcoid. One of the commonest mani-
festations of sarcoid is bilateral sym-
metrical enlargement of hilar lymph
nodes. Erythema nodosum, low
grade fever and polyarthritis are very
common initial findings.

b Further investigations are as follows.

• Biopsy of skin lesions. Showed a nonspecific inflammatory response. (In
patients with sarcoid, the non caseat-
ing epithelioid granulomata usually
seen in the typical erythema nodosum
skin lesions are diagnostic.)

• Kveim test. This is a useful diagnostic
procedure, providing that a potent
antigen (obtained from human sarcoid tissue) is used. Its disadvantage
is the 4–6 weeks required before the
resulting skin nodule can be biopsied.
In this case, the Kveim test was
negative.

• Mantoux reaction. Skin sensitivity to
tuberculin is depressed or absent so
that a strongly positive test virtually
excludes sarcoid.

Grey case 21 (Part 2 c–e)

c Hodgkin's disease. The patient now exhibits typical systemic symptoms, although the absence of cervical or axillary lymphadenopathy is unusual. Skin rashes in Hodgkin's disease are almost always nonspecific reactions occurring in up to 30% of patients. Histological evidence, usually Reed–Sternberg cells, occur in only about 3% of these patients.

d CT scanning of thorax and abdomen. This showed enlargement of multiple intra-abdominal lymph nodes, including para-aortic and retroperitoneal groups, and confirmed the clinical findings of bilateral hilar adenopathy and splenomegaly. Bone marrow aspirate and trephine were both normal, giving useful information for staging of the disease.

e Histological diagnosis is more difficult when a peripheral lymph node is unavailable for biopsy. Closed biopsy of mediastinal masses is potentially dangerous and sometimes associated with excessive bleeding from vascular lesions. Open biopsy of the mediastinum should be considered, but, in this case, the diagnosis was established by splenectomy. The para-aortic lymph nodes were also infiltrated with disease.

Grey case 21 (Part 3 f, g)

f Nodular sclerosing (NS) Hodgkin's disease. Mediastinal disease in young women is very likely to be NS. (This is especially so when disease is confined to the mediastinum.)

g Multidrug chemotherapy (e.g. MOPP). If the mediastinal disease is 'bulky' (>33% of the thoracic width), radiotherapy to the mass should be included at some stage of treatment in view of the relatively high relapse rate in patients treated only with chemotherapy.

Grey case 22

a Bone marrow and CSF show active haemophagocytosis by histiocytes.

b In view of the clinical features, laboratory results, family history, and the striking morphological features, the diagnosis of haemophagocytic lymphohistiocytosis (HLH) can be made. Despite this being a first child, the consanguinity of parents suggests a familial disorder. This condition was previously known as familial erythrophagocytic lymphohistiocytosis (FEL).

c Despite not being a true malignant disease, this condition runs a miserable course and requires aggressive treatment with chemotherapeutic agents. Where possible bone marrow transplantation is associated with the best long-term survival. This child was treated with VP16 (etoposide) and methylprednisolone resulting in a marked improvement in his condition. He was extubated and returned to the ward. A further two courses of VP16 were given. Tissue typing of parents and child revealed that the father was a full class I and class II HLA match. He proceeded to allogeneic bone marrow transplantation with busulphan and cyclophosphamide conditioning. Despite being the first child of this couple it has to be assumed that this is a familial disorder, and therefore it is extremely important that these parents have genetic counselling.

Grey case 23 (Part 1 a)

a Investigations required are:
- examination of blood film;
- DCT;
- serum B_{12} and folate levels;
- reticulocyte count;
- bone marrow examination;
- autoantibody screen;
- serum electrophoresis.

Grey case 23 (Part 2 b, c)

b The most likely diagnosis is auto-immune haemolytic anaemia. This may lead to slight splenomegaly. The blood film was not entirely typical. However, it did show some spherocytes. Reticulocyte count was raised, as was the bilirubin. The megaloblastic changes were presumed to be secondary to folate deficiency, although serum folate levels were normal. It may have been preferable in this case to measure red cell folate.

c The usual management would be high-dose steroids, for example prednisolone 60 mg daily, and folic acid 5 mg daily.

Grey case 23 (Part 3 d)

d It should be possible to crossmatch using autoabsorbed serum to provide compatible blood.

Grey case 23 (Part 4 e–g)

e The findings of erythroid hypoplasia in the bone marrow indicate a diagnosis of pure red cell aplasia.

f This may be caused by drugs, including azathioprine, infections, autoimmune disorders, or can be associated with a thymoma.

g Immediate further management includes stopping azathioprine, but continuing steroids and red cell transfusion. Investigations would include autoantibody screen, infection screen including parvovirus B19, chest radiograph, and CT scan of the thorax.

Grey case 23 (Part 5 h)

h Patients who have undergone splenectomy are prone to overwhelming sepsis, particularly pneumococcal infections. It is important that they receive Pneumovax pre-operatively and advisable that the patients take penicillin prophylactically for an indefinite period of time. If the patient is allergic to penicillin, erythromycin may be substituted.

Grey case 23 (Part 6 i, j)

i Thymoma. CT scan of the thorax showed a calcified soft tissue mass in the anterior mediastinum with no hilar lymphadenopathy.

j The patient underwent a mediastinotomy and thymectomy. The histology proved to be benign, but the patient remained transfusion-dependent. Other therapeutic measures that may be tried include the use of anti-lymphocyte globulin and cyclosporin A. In this case cyclosporin A was prescribed, which resulted in an elevation of the Hb. The patient maintains a Hb of approximately 10 g/dl on cyclosporin A 50 mg b.d. with no renal impairment.

Grey case 24 (Part 1 a–e)

a Myelofibrosis.
b A splenic infarct.
c Chronic myeloid leukaemia.
  Myelofibrosis is more likely because of the patient's age, the relatively low WCC, and the prominent red cell changes. The basophilia could occur in either condition.
d A splenic rub.
e Cytogenetics on blood or bone marrow.

Grey case 24 (Part 2 f, g)

f Ph⁻, BCR⁺ chronic myeloid leukaemia (about 5% of CML patients are genuinely Ph⁻ and the majority will produce the 8.5 kb BCR-ABL mRNA and the 210 kd BCR-ABL protein. These patients usually have a normal karyotype or an abnormality involving chromosome 9 band q34, with clinical and laboratory features that are indistinguishable from those of Ph⁺ CML patients).
g Busulphan or hydroxyurea. Alpha-interferon may be considered, but should used with care in the elderly because of its potential side-effects.

Grey case 24 (Part 3 h, i)

h The differential diagnosis is:
● intracerebral oozing of blood secondary to marked thrombocytopenia;
● blast cell transformation presenting in the CNS, which should be considered in view of the progression of the karyotype, the re-emergence of basophilia and the atypical lymphoid cells. Additional chromosomal changes, especially the Ph chromosome and the isochromosome 17 are often associated with or precede blast transformation, which usually occurs in blood and marrow, but can occur at other sites, especially the CNS.
i CT scan of the intracranial contents was normal. Lumbar puncture revealed macroscopically normal CSF, which contained large numbers of CD19-positive leukaemic blasts, suggesting a CNS transformation to ALL.

Grey case 25 (Part 1 a–c)

a This man apparently has an element of chronic bronchitis and emphysema and atherosclerosis due in part to his relatively high cigarette consumption. His Hb is at the upper end of the normal range. The ESR is raised. The WCC is high normal and the platelets significantly raised. His haematological changes could be secondary to inflammatory changes, e.g. lung and gangrenous toes, and hypoxia (along with carboxyhaemoglobin). It is unclear whether he might have relative or stress polycythaemia, or true polycythaemia which could be either secondary to mild hypoxia or a myeloproliferative disorder. The platelet count is higher than would be anticipated from a mild basal chest infection and a single gangrenous toe. The presence of target cells on the blood film suggest a degree of hepatic dysfunction (secondary to alcohol excess) or hyposplenism (as a result of asymptomatic infarction due to possible essential thrombocythaemia).

b In summary the differential diagnosis is:
- myeloproliferative disorder;
- relative polycythaemia;
- secondary polycythaemia due to mild hypoxia (and carboxyhaemoglobinaemia) caused by chronic bronchitis and emphysema;
- atherosclerosis.

c Further investigations indicated are red cell mass and plasma volume, bleeding time, platelet aggregation studies, abdominal ultrasound to assess liver and spleen size and texture, and uric acid.

Grey case 25 (Part 2 d, e)

d The results are most in keeping with the diagnosis of essential thrombocythaemia as the red cell mass and plasma volume are normal. The bleeding time is sometimes prolonged in this condition and aggregation to adrenaline may be absent. The small spleen (due to silent infarction) is in keeping with a diagnosis of essential thrombocythaemia. The marginally raised urate is a feature of myeloproliferative disorders.

e He should be strongly encouraged to give up smoking. Aspirin 300 mg daily is often very effective as a platelet inhibitor in this condition and may lead to a marked improvement in the toe ischaemia. The platelet count should be reduced; hydroxyurea is very effective and could prove a useful drug for long-term management. Once the platelet count approaches normal values, radiophosphorus could be considered.

Grey case 26 (Part 1 a, b)

a The bone marrow shows dysplastic changes and is hypercellular. This, in conjunction with the peripheral pancytopenia is entirely consistent with a diagnosis of myelodysplastic syndrome.

b The most appropriate treatment for a patient of this age at this stage of disease is platelet concentrates, antibiotics for infection, and transfusion with packed cells when the patient becomes symptomatic.

Grey case 26 (Part 2 c, d)

c The history of dark urine suggests haemoglobinuria and intravascular haemolysis.
• Tests for urinary haemosiderin proved positive.
• The direct Coomb's test was negative.
• Haptoglobins were decreased at less than 0.5 g/l.
• Renal function was normal.
• Liver function tests were normal.

• Reticulocyte count was increased at 99 x 10^9/l.

d If a patient presents with intravascular haemolysis, pancytopenia, and vague abdominal pains, a diagnosis of paroxysmal haemoglobinuria must be considered. PNH may arise in a dysplastic marrow. In this patient, both the Hams test and sucrose lysis test were positive.

Grey case 26 (Part 3 e–g)

e It was calculated that this lady had been transfused more than 150 units of red cells since her initial presentation. Although there will have been some loss of iron from the body during the episodes of intravascular haemolysis, it was believed that she was suffering from a transfusional siderosis, which had affected her liver and her joints, giving her chondrocalcinosis. Another possibility for the abdominal pain and jaundice would have been an episode of post-transfusional hepatitis C.

f Further useful tests would be:
• serum ferritin, which was elevated at 4477 µg/l (15–300 µg/l);
• serum iron, which was 28 µmol/l (10–35 µmol/l);
• total iron binding capacity, which was 28.5 µmol/l (35–70 µmol/l);
• urea and electrolytes, which were normal.
  Both the transferrin saturation (i.e. serum iron/TIBC), and serum ferritin suggest that this lady is suffering from iron overload.

g Venesection is inappropriate and so treatment with intravenous or subcutaneous desferrioxamine with oral vitamin C would be useful.

Grey case 27

a The pericardial fluid and bone marrow contain an abnormal clone of cells demonstrated on cytogenetics. The immunophenotype indicates a mixed lymphoid population of cells only. The karyotype shows hypodyploidy, but is not specific for any individual malignancy. The marrow slide shows blast cells with low nucleocytoplasmic ratio and prominent nucleoli. The clinical and laboratory features suggest a haematological malignancy, probably acute lymphoblastic leukaemia or stage IV non-Hodgkin's lymphoma.

b Cytochemistry and immunophenotype are required on the marrow sample. Other investigations should include abdominal ultrasound, chest radiograph, and lumbar puncture for CSF cell count and cytospin. In this case blast immunophenotype indicated common ALL, and repeat marrow after one week showed 80% blasts. Hypodiploidy is a recognised feature in ALL and carries a poor prognosis.

Grey case 28

a Diagnoses include thrombotic thrombocytopenic purpura (TTP), haemolytic uraemic syndrome (HUS) and early DIC secondary to septicaemia arising from the retained dead fetus. TTP is most likely particularly as it is associated with pregnancy. It must have been present for some considerable period for her Hb to have fallen to such a low level and for a marked reticulocyte count to have emerged. HUS is less likely because the urea is normal and she has not had any preceding diarrhoea. It is just possible that she has early DIC secondary to pelvic or uterine infection.

b A D and C to evacuate the uterus must be urgently arranged. A transfusion of red cells should be started to raise her Hb. Daily plasma exchange with replacement by fresh frozen plasma should be started immediately after the D and C. Such treatment should be continued until the platelet count rises substantially and the haemolysis diminishes. This can be monitored by serial reticulocyte counts and plasma LDH estimations.

c There is a distinct possibility that it will recur during a subsequent pregnancy. During the current pregnancy the TTP had started early and led to the death of the fetus. If she decided to have a further pregnancy the risk to mother and fetus must be explained. If she became pregnant she should immediately have a FBC, reticulocytes and LDH estimation. She could be started on daily aspirin. If any signs of TTP begin to develop, regular plasma exchange should be started. Such a programme may control the process in pregnancy.

Index

Note: page numbers for both questions and answers are given, with answer page numbers in bold. Page numbers in *italics* refer to figures.

chronic skin, 83, **116**
granulocytes, left shifted, *81*, **114**

haematoma, *14*, 17, **32**, **34**, 77, **111**
    circulatory inhibitor of coagulation system,
        77, **111**
    of the psoas, *24*, **39**
haematopoiesis, extramedullary, *82*, **114**, *115*
haemochromatosis, 78, **113**
haemoglobin electrophoresis, *45*, **62**
haemoglobinopathy screen, *45*, **62**
haemoglobinuria, 102, **130**
    paroxysmal cold, *41*, **59**, *92*, **122**
    paroxysmal nocturnal (PNH), 83, **116**
haemolysis
    autoimmune, *44*, **61**
    chronic oxidative intravascular, *19*, **35**
    intravascular, *91–2*, 102, **122**, **130**
    risk with G6PD deficiency, *48*, **64**
haemolytic anaemia, 7, **28**
    acute warm, *44*, **61**
    microangiopathic, *25*, **39**
haemolytic disease of the newborn, 89, **120**
    ABO, *92–3*, **122–3**
haemolytic uraemic syndrome (HUS), *25*, **39**,
    73, **107**
haemophagocytic lymphohistiocytosis (HLH),
    15, **33**, *96*, **125–6**
haemophagocytosis, *15*, *23*, **32**, **38**
haemophilia, *24*, **39**
    acquired, 77, **111**, **112**
    congenital, 112
haemophilia A
    carrier, *46*, **63**
    intragenic factor VIII BclII polymorphic site
        alleles, *49*, **64**
    obligate carriers, *49*, **64**
    severe, *49*, **64**
hairy cell leukaemia (HCL), *52*, **66**
Ham's acidified serum lysis test, 83, 102, **116**, **130**
heart valve
    haemolysis, 7, **28**
    leaking prosthetic, 7, **28**
Heinz bodies, *19*, **35**
heparin therapy, 94, **124**
hepatic and renal failure, combined, *14*, **32**
hepatic veno-occlusive disease of the liver, 75,
    110
hepatitis, alcoholic, 79, **113**
hepatitis B, 75, **109**
    decompensated, *44*, **61**
hepatitis C, *44*, **61**
hepatocellular carcinoma, 79, **113**
hepatoma, 79, **113**
hepatomegaly, 80, 81
hepatosplenomegaly, *15*, *22*, *24*, **32**, **37**, **38**, 50, **66**
    ALL, 103, **131**
    Down's syndrome, 76, **110**
    multi-system disease, *88*, **119**
hereditary persistence of fetal haemoglobin
    (HPFH), *50*, **65**

hereditary spherocytosis (HS), *17*, **34**, *53*, **67**
histiocytes, *15*, **32**
    haemophagocytosis, *96*, **125**
histiocytosis X, *88*, **119**
Hodgkin's disease, nodular sclerosing, 95, **125**
Howell–Jolly bodies, *9*, **29**
humerus spontaneous fracture, 50, **65**
hydroxyurea, 80, 90, **114**, **121**
    CML treatment, *99–100*, **128**
hyperleucocytosis, 71, **105**
hypersplenia, *82*, **114**
hyposplenism, *9*, **29**
hysterectomy, lupus anticoagulants, *56*, **68**

IgG
    levels in leucoerythroblastic anaemia, *84*, **117**
    paraprotein, 8, **28**
immunoglobulin, intravenous therapy, *85*, 93,
    118, **123**
immunosuppression, aplastic anaemia, *47*, **63**
infant monosomy 7 syndrome, *10*, **27**
infection, atypical, 93, **123**
infectious mononucleosis, *41*, **59**
intracerebral bleeding, 71, **105**
intrathoracic primary tumour, *18*, **35**
iron overload, 102, **130**
ischaemia, toe, 100, **129**

juvenile chronic myeloid leukaemia (JCML),
    10, **29**, *80*, *81*, **114**
juvenile myeloproliferative disorders, *10*, **29**

kala-azar, 93, **123**
Kell phenotype, 89, **120**
Kostmann's syndrome, *9*, **29**
Kveim tests, 95, **124**

Langerhan cell histiocytosis, *88*, **119**
lecithin/sphingomyelin ratio, *89*, **120**
Leishman–Donovan bodies, 93, **123**
Leishmaniasis, 93, **123**
leukaemoid reaction in neonatal period, 76, **111**
liposomal Amphoterocin, 93, **123**
liver
    chronic disease, 78, **112**
    dysfunction, *15*, **32**
lupus anticoagulants, *56*, **68**
lymph node
    basophilic cells, *23*, **37**
    enlargement, 95, **125**
lymphadenopathy, *22*, *24*, **37**, **38**, *84*, **117**
    multi-system disease, *88*, **119**
lymphoblastic lymphoma, T cell, *23*, **37**
lymphocyte stress test, 20, **36**
lymphoma
    follicular, *51*, **66**
    T cell, *51*, **66**

134